# The Mental Health Contagion™
### *Navigating Yourself Through a Loved One's Mental Well-Being Decline*

## Yvette Murray

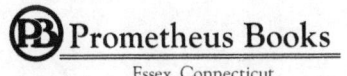
Essex, Connecticut

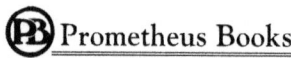 Prometheus Books

An imprint of The Globe Pequot Publishing Group, Inc.
64 South Main Street
Essex, CT 06426
www.GlobePequot.com

Copyright © 2025 by Yvette Murray

*All rights reserved.* No part of this book may be reproduced in any form or by any electronic or mechanical means, including information storage and retrieval systems, without written permission from the publisher, except by a reviewer who may quote passages in a review.

British Library Cataloguing in Publication Information available

**Library of Congress Cataloging-in-Publication Data available**
ISBN 978-1-4930-9094-5 (paper)
ISBN 978-1-4930-9095-2 (electronic)

*This book is dedicated to my mother—my inspiration, my cheerleader—and to my father, who was the backbone for all of us.*

## DISCLAIMER

**Please be aware that some content in this book may be triggering, including discussions of suicide, so please be gentle with yourself as you read. If you are in distress, you can call or text 988 at any time. If it is an emergency, call 911 or go to your local emergency department.**

Neither the publisher nor the author offers professional advice to the reader in this book. The ideas and suggestions provided are not intended as a substitute for seeking professional guidance.

In order to maintain their anonymity, in some instances the author has changed the names of individuals. The views expressed by the author are in no way a reflection of her clients, affiliates, or associations.

# Contents

Foreword by Kevin B. Murray . . . . . . . . . . . . . . . . . vii

Chapter 1: The Mental Health Contagion™ Risk . . . . . . . . 1
Chapter 2: How Do You Recognize the Signs/Symptoms of
          Mental Health Decline? . . . . . . . . . . . . . . . . . 9
Chapter 3: The Four As: Awareness, Acknowledgment,
          Acceptance, and Action = Change . . . . . . . . . . . . 39
Chapter 4: "How Do I Make It All Better?" . . . . . . . . . . . . 59
Chapter 5: Help Me Help You Help Me . . . . . . . . . . . . 69
Chapter 6: Handling Unhealthy Behaviors and
          Setting Boundaries . . . . . . . . . . . . . . . . . . . 89
Chapter 7: Avoiding Burnout . . . . . . . . . . . . . . . . . 107
Chapter 8: Cultivating Resilience . . . . . . . . . . . . . . . 127

Epilogue: Climbing Your Mountain . . . . . . . . . . . . . . 147
Acknowledgments . . . . . . . . . . . . . . . . . . . . . . 155
About the Author . . . . . . . . . . . . . . . . . . . . . . 159

# Foreword

## *by Kevin B. Murray*

As Yvette's father I have been navigating a loved one's mental well-being decline firsthand since the early 1970s. I can validate the efficacy of the methods cited in *The Mental Health Contagion*™ for a real family.

I'm grateful to have the opportunity to reflect on and introduce this roadmap for you, the significant other, family member, friend, colleague, and/or caregiver. I only wish I had access to its practical advice at the start of my journey.

This work focuses on the well-being of those who are struggling or overwhelmed from trying to cope with the challenges involved in caring for loved ones. The author explains the simple truth: While dealing with serious emotional issues and caring for loved ones, there is an inherent susceptibility to contracting the contagion of mental and physical decline ourselves.

Yvette speaks her truth and explains some of the most common mental health problems and disorders, as well as demystifying the signs and symptoms of a mental well-being decline. The book homes in on practical tools and effective examples designed to help readers recognize and ward off mental and physical decline in themselves and others. The author also paves many ways to surmount co-occurring mental and physical challenges, including building resilience to achieve successful outcomes.

Yes, mental health decline can be contagious in both mind and body. The stigma surrounding mental health issues has also contributed to the contagion. This book incorporates many effective lessons and resources to help you remember to care for yourself and avoid your own physical and mental decline while navigating your way through a loved one's or someone else's mental health issues.

We very easily overlook the fact that when problems arise, accompanied by continuous exposure to stressful situations, breakdowns can result that impair our coping mechanisms and ability to function properly, further leading to anxiety and frustration. As a response to stress, anxiety can produce phobias and manifest worrisome physical symptoms. The more challenging circumstances become, the higher the risk to our own mental well-being. This book addresses the need for proper checks and balances, as well as preventative measures along the way.

In sum, this book addresses the importance of taking care of ourselves, managing the challenges associated with physical and mental decline, and understanding that everyone benefits when we are rested and physically and mentally healthy. Yvette delves right into her "juicy bits" about self-care, which aren't just what we do when we're spent or on the verge of breaking down. We must be proactive about it and determine what we personally need to build our resilience. Yvette invites you on a test drive on the road of her own Mental Health Contagion™ journey to help master the traffic lights and roundabouts. The book is written in a pragmatic, inspiring, and conversational style that's rich in inspiration, wit, and wisdom.

This foreword serves as testimony to the legacy of all those who have dedicated their lives and competencies to the medical-clinical and therapeutical caring professions, in particular to the mother of the author. You will read more about her through Yvette's experiences. Along with her own mental health challenges, Margaret faced the ordeal of her immigration to Canada in 1967, and after graduating in 1973 worked as a nurse specializing in psychiatric nursing and post-graduate community mental health—all while raising a family of four children.

Margaret Murray's pioneering therapies and solutions for coping with stress and despair were featured in the *Report/Health* supplement in the May 20, 1980, edition of the *Ottawa Citizen*. Karen Moser, *Citizen* staff writer, wrote: "Nepean Police are a little less edgy since the British born Psychiatric Nurse and Relaxation Therapist arrived on the scene." Margaret also exerted her calming influence on Ottawa Airport's air traffic controllers, bank managers, lawyers, housewives, and teenagers through private practice, online radio, and in television mental health segments.

Suffice it to say that Yvette Murray, the author of *The Mental Health Contagion*™, clearly followed in her mother's footsteps. Yvette has traveled worldwide and brings into context her own experiences navigating a loved one's mental well-being decline, along with the advice and counsel of her many professional colleagues and friends in various fields of therapeutic care. Enjoy the ride and read.

Chapter One

# The Mental Health Contagion™ Risk

"Phew! He's gone to work. I can come out of the closet," I thought as I heard the pitter patter of my dad's feet climbing down the stairs, followed by the sound of the side door closing.

I tiptoed out of my room and opened my parents' bedroom door. "I'm here!" I announced, giving my mother quite a shock.

I was supposed to be at school, but I had my own plan of staying home with my mom to keep her company.

I didn't know it then, but I now realize that my eight-year-old mind believed I was saving my mom. If I stayed by her side, I could take care of her and protect her from herself. I frequently came down with a sore throat and lethargy. I'd miss weeks of school at a time, all in the name of manifesting reasons to stay home with Mom.

My mother—Margaret, Mags, or Maggie—had been diagnosed with bipolar disorder that was sometimes left untreated. At times during my childhood, she was hospitalized, and she attempted suicide more than once. As you can imagine this was very traumatic for me. Each family member experienced this crisis differently. We did our best to keep up with the family routines—going to school, meals, etc.—however, the emotional toll and fear of the unknown was felt throughout the whole family. She was a psychiatric nurse who was passionate about helping others with mental illness. Meanwhile, mental health problems ran in our family, so there were others among us who were struggling.

Certainly, for me as a little girl and into adulthood, my mother's illness was life-changing in more ways than one. For one thing, the belief that I could somehow save my mother stuck with me decades after I stayed home from school with her—until her dying day. So I come by my desire to help you navigate your own loved one's mental well-being decline naturally. I no longer have illusions about saving anyone, but both personally and professionally, I have learned a great deal about how to handle such a situation.

Interestingly, as I began to write this book and meet with my editor, I got that all-too-familiar sore throat and lethargy again—just like in my childhood. I'm amazed at the connection between the mind and body. When something manifests physically, it can create a risk to our mental health, and when our mind experiences symptoms, it can directly impact us physically. For example, the symptoms of a panic attack are eerily like that of a heart attack. In her book, *Heal Your Body*, Louise Hay wrote that a sore throat can be a symptom of not speaking your truth.

Unlike when I was a child, I'm now able to speak my truth in this book as someone with years of experience in the mental health field. I also know all too well the importance of self-care while navigating through someone else's mental health decline. And this book is primarily about making sure that you care for yourself, no matter how challenging your circumstances may become. You see, mental health decline is contagious.

## The Mental Health Contagion™

Just like we all have physical health, we all have mental health. No one is exempt from experiencing a mental health problem, crisis, and/or disorder. And even though mental health isn't transmitted like a virus, we are still susceptible to feeling its effects from someone else. Someone can have an anxiety disorder, for example, and it can create anxiety in others around them. Their symptoms can affect us and put our own mental health at risk. That risk is higher without the proper support, tools, and preventative measures. This book is designed to give you the tools, preventative measures, and resources for support that you need to guard against your own mental well-being decline.

The stigma surrounding mental health issues has also contributed to the contagion, as well as the lack of self-care among caregivers. I recently came back from a trip to the United Kingdom to visit my mother's sister, who is now ninety-five years old. She shared with me that mental health was a "dirty word" and wasn't spoken about when she was growing up. "Your mother should have gotten help for her mental illness when signs of it showed up in her youth," she said. Instead of actual help, when they discovered my mother on the stairs almost catatonic in emotional distress, her father asked my aunt to "go make Margaret smile."

Luckily, today, society has more of a collective recognition that mental health issues are at an all-time high and that they need to be addressed by professionals. The more open we become about discussing mental well-being, the better off we will all be, and that includes the need to take good care of ourselves when we struggle with someone who is declining.

Mental health awareness educational programs have become readily available to help reduce the stigma and recognize the signs/symptoms of someone with a mental health disorder, crisis, or problem. I'm a facilitator of the Mental Health First Aid certification, an evidence-based program available in more than thirty countries around the world. This program has been instrumental in opening the dialogue and demystifying mental health. During my keynotes, courses, and corporate engagements, people also seek support on how to navigate themselves through the challenging, sometimes heart-wrenching circumstances they experience with someone who is living with a mental illness. In my work, I have seen the Mental Health Contagion™ in countless situations, where people don't have the tools they need to prevent it. That's why I have felt compelled to write this book.

## Self-Care

I used to believe it was selfish to take care of yourself, especially when someone else had it "worse." "How could I possibly think of myself at a time like this?" I thought. But after being surrounded during many of my formative and adult years by loved ones going through a mental health decline, I discovered firsthand that self-care is imperative.

In fact, I'm so convinced of the importance of self-care that I was once prepared to get arrested! Prior to the COVID-19 lockdowns, I would regularly travel to my hometown for family time and make a point of visiting a spa with Linda, my best friend of several decades.

This was our time to catch up, de-stress, giggle, and take care of our mind, body, and spirit.

Fast forward to the day before the COVID-19 lockdown was lifted. The spa was a short distance between provincial borders, and crossing the border was for essential purposes only. As I approached the Stop sign just around the corner from the spa, there were several police cars asking each driver if they had a legitimate reason to cross the border. With my mask on and window rolled down, the officer asked my purpose and where I was going. "I'm heading to the spa with the purpose of self-care," I said. I showed him my frontline worker mental health facilitator identification. "In order for me to be of service, I need this trip to the spa," I emphasized. There was a pause, then a chuckle from him. He took one look in my eyes, and I believe he felt my conviction. In my mind, they would need to handcuff me before I would *not* go to that spa! He smiled and waved me on.

At that moment, I acknowledged my own dedication to self and showed by example my commitment to "walk my talk." The experience also gave me hope that society is starting to recognize the need for self-care.

It's when we care for ourselves that we're best equipped to manage the challenges we face, and others in our life benefit the most when we're rested and healthy both physically and mentally. Yet, we don't have to defend or justify our need to be good to ourselves. Beyond all the excellent reasons for self-care, *we deserve it just because we do.*

It's true that when others aren't used to seeing us do things for ourselves, they might get their feathers ruffled. I sometimes heard comments like, "It must be nice to have the time to do that" or "Some people are lucky." However, when they saw how I showed up healthier, more present, and stronger in relationships, at work, in my community, and at home, comments shifted to, "I want some of what *you're* having!"

The other day, my brother called to say, "I did an 'Yvette' today."

"What's an 'Yvette?'" I asked.

He reminded me of the conversation we had earlier in the day when I mentioned the importance of self-care. Therefore, he (and others in my circle) now refer to such actions as an 'Yvette.'" I couldn't be more pleased to be their role model in this respect.

But if you think self-care is all about pampering, bubble baths, and spas, think again. Although these can provide support, there are many other self-care tools that also have a proven track record. Throughout this book, I will share these tools and insights on how self-care will make a difference in helping you with a wide range of mental health risk factors. We will go much more in depth to cover what you need to preserve your own mental health when you're faced with someone who is challenged by theirs.

## Is This Book for You?

Do you feel lost about how to support your loved one, friend, or colleague who is going through a mental well-being decline, all while you feel yourself standing in quicksand, getting sucked into a dark hole?

The chances are high you've picked up this book for support and answers that you may have felt too embarrassed, ashamed, or guilty to ask. Perhaps you are feeling vulnerable, uneasy, or even fearful of the unknown. You might be walking on eggshells while supporting someone you care about who is suffering.

As an international mental health speaker and advocate, I've been in front of thousands of audiences, clients, and communities worldwide, and these are some of the most common questions I've been asked:

- What if I say the wrong thing?
- Are my actions or words causing them to be this way?
- Am I in danger?
- How can I be there for someone without compromising my own psychological safety and basic needs?
- What do I do with my emotions through this experience?
- How do I carry on and not lose myself in their illness?
- How do I not get a mental illness myself?
- Is it normal to feel angry at my loved one, even though I know what they are going through?
- How can I help someone if they don't want to help themselves?
- Do I stay or leave?

If you struggle to find answers to questions like these, this book is definitely for you. It will provide you with many strategies to make sure you preserve your own mental wellness as you interact with and serve the person you love.

After having experienced this firsthand and then working with hundreds of other people who are going through it, I know there is a way through the darkness, despair, and hopelessness. You'll read relatable stories in the chapters that follow, as you learn how to make the situation better for you, even if you can't make it better for your loved one.

Here is what we'll cover as you continue reading:

*Chapter 2—How Do You Recognize the Signs/Symptoms of Mental Health Decline?* While this isn't an invitation to diagnose anyone, it will help you see the usual signs and symptoms that accompany mental wellness decline.

*Chapter 3—The Four As: Awareness, Acknowledgment, Acceptance, and Action = Change.* You will learn how these four As can help you move from victimhood to healthy action that can bring about positive change.

*Chapter 4—"How Do I Make It All Better?"* You may want to do all you can to help your loved one get better, but in doing so, you could inadvertently make the situation worse. This chapter will show you what to watch for to make sure you are handling everything in a way that will benefit all involved.

*Chapter 5—Help Me Help You Help Me.* Sometimes, the only way to know what someone else needs is to let them tell you, rather than make assumptions about what you think they "should" need. Learn the questions you can ask and more.

*Chapter 6—Handling Unhealthy Behaviors and Setting Boundaries.* It's vital that caregivers and loved ones learn to set boundaries when dealing with someone in a mental wellness decline. It's perhaps the most important aspect of self-care.

*Chapter 7—Avoiding Burnout.* Is there a way to avoid burning out when dealing with someone who is challenging and possibly demanding? Yes!

*Chapter 8—Cultivating Resilience.* One of the most important ways to practice self-care is to learn how to become stronger. Discover how to manage your emotions and do what I call "deadheading" your life.

*Epilogue.* In these final words, I will bring the information you've learned throughout the book into a cohesive message that I hope will help you feel more encouraged and better able to handle what comes.

Each chapter will include what I call "Juicy Bits"—short pieces of wisdom from the chapter. You will also find a few exercises in the book to help you apply the tools to your own situation.

Trust that there is a way to navigate through this with more dignity, calm, and balance. I'll be your tour guide as you read these pages. Here's your life jacket. . . .

CHAPTER TWO

# How Do You Recognize the Signs/Symptoms of Mental Health Decline?

WHEN I TRAVEL TO GIVE MENTAL HEALTH KEYNOTE SPEECHES, I LIKE to connect with any friends and family who live in the area. So on a recent trip, I met a friend for coffee.

We got to talking about the writing of this book, and my friend disclosed his feelings of guilt because he has a great life, while his brother, who struggles with mental illness, lives "on the streets." My friend said he felt shame, fear, hopelessness, and anxiety about the situation. But he had an "aha!" moment when he saw a therapist to help him with these feelings. The therapist explained the symptoms of his brother's mental health disorder, which caused a weight to be lifted off my friend's shoulders.

This reminds me of the slogan spoken in the London subway intercom system: "See it, Say it, and Sort it." It constantly reminds passengers that if they see something that could be a safety risk, they should speak to a subway employee so that it can be sorted out.

There is healing in seeing the signs and symptoms, speaking about them, and taking action to support ourselves and others. In this chapter, my intention is to demystify some of the most common mental health problems and disorders. This guidance isn't meant to be used for diagnoses however. It's simply offered to help you recognize the signs and symptoms of mental well-being decline. You may even recognize some of these within yourself!

As I've said, when we're around someone with serious emotional issues, it's easy to become susceptible to mental health decline ourselves. Therefore, we can watch for these same signs and symptoms in ourselves and ward off any issues before they become bigger. Early intervention is key, so it's important to stay aware and attentive.

## The Hereditary Element

Scientists have long recognized that many psychiatric disorders tend to run in families, suggesting potential genetic roots. Such disorders include bipolar disorder, major depression, and schizophrenia. Although there's some risk of a genetic link with mental illness, I won't focus on this. The signs and symptoms remain the same regardless of the source of the problem.

### MENTAL HEALTH *DISORDERS* VS. MENTAL HEALTH *PROBLEMS*

According to the World Health Organization, "a mental disorder is characterized by a clinically significant disturbance in an individual's cognition, emotional regulation, or behavior. It is usually associated with distress or impairment in important areas of functioning."[1] A mental health disorder is a diagnosable illness.

Mental health and substance use problems affect people from all walks and stages of life. Mental illnesses can impact many areas of an individual's life, how they show up in relationships, in their community, and at work, as well as their ability to manage their finances. The effects can be felt by anyone in contact with the individual, and these symptoms are costly to them, their family, their community, and the health care system at large.

There's a misguided belief, however, that when someone is living with a mental health disorder, they can't work, contribute to society, or have a meaningful, healthy, functioning life. This isn't true. Many mental health and substance use problems can be time-limited, so people can resume their lives as before if they have the right treatment, support system, and

---

1. World Health Organization, "Mental Disorders," June 8, 2022, accessed November 1, 2024, https://www.who.int/news-room/fact-sheets/detail/mental-disorders.

tools. Just as someone diagnosed with diabetes can live a healthy functioning life with proper intervention, or those reaching middle age can sharpen their vision with reading glasses, it is possible for those living with mental health issues to live a satisfying, hopeful, and contributing life, even when there may be ongoing limitations as result of the mental health problems and illnesses.

As I teach in the Mental First Aid course, a mental health or substance use "problem" is a broader term that includes both illnesses and symptoms of illnesses that may not be severe enough to warrant the diagnosis of a "disorder."

The word *problem* covers a wider range of mental health or substance use concerns, from the worries we all experience as part of everyday life to mental health or substance use "disorders" that more severely impact someone's ability to carry out daily life activities or maintain relationships.

In this chapter, I have highlighted some of the evidence-based signs and symptoms that are commonly written about. I've referenced various sources, and many of these signs and symptoms are also outlined in the *Mental Health First Aid Reference Guide*. Please note that this list is not exhaustive, and it's the information we know as of today. As times evolve, we evolve, so we're continually learning and discovering more about the complexities of mental health. For example, years ago, it was believed that schizophrenia was caused by the patient's poor relationship with their mother, or living in poverty. As we know today, this isn't true.

For some of you, defining mental health problems and disorders will be new, while for others, it will be a refresher or affirmation of what your loved one may be going through. Remember, however, that the following information isn't for the purposes of diagnosing anyone!

## PROBLEMS/DISORDERS
### *Agoraphobia*
There is a common belief that agoraphobia is the fear of going outside. In fact, a person with agoraphobia experiences anxiety that occurs when they're in a public or crowded place. The fear is that there's no escape and that help won't be accessible. They believe it will be embarrassing or difficult to get away from the place if a panic attack or other symptom

occurs. Although agoraphobia can occur without panic attacks, this is less common. (See Anxiety below and Panic Attacks on page 20.)

*Anxiety*

Everyone experiences anxiety at some point in their life. Occasional anxiety is a normal part of life. Many people worry about things such as health, money, or family problems. But anxiety disorders involve more than temporary worry or fear. For people with an anxiety disorder, the anxiety doesn't go away and can get worse over time. I personally feel anxiety the most when I'm caught up in worries about what *might* happen, even if it's unlikely. People might describe anxiety as feeling stressed, uptight, nervous, frazzled, worried, tense, or hassled.

Anxiety can, of course, be useful if it helps us avoid dangerous situations and solve everyday problems. But some people are more likely than others to react with anxiety when they feel threatened even if there isn't any real danger.

Anxiety can vary in severity from mild uneasiness to a terrifying panic attack that makes us feel like we're having a heart attack. It can also vary in how long it lasts, from a few moments to many years. Anxiety problems differ from normal anxiety in the following ways:

- More severe and intense
- Last longer
- Interfere with daily activities, work, and relationships

*Signs and Symptoms of Anxiety*

Some physical symptoms of anxiety are:

- Pounding heart, chest pain, rapid heartbeat, blushing
- Rapid, shallow breathing and shortness of breath
- Dizziness, headache, sweating, tingling, and numbness
- Choking, dry mouth, stomach pains, nausea, vomiting, and diarrhea
- Muscle aches and pains (especially neck, shoulders, and back)
- Restlessness, tremors, and shaking

Anxiety can also affect people's thinking, behavior, and physical well-being, as follows:

**Thinking.** People living with anxiety may experience their mind racing or going blank, decreased concentration and memory, indecisiveness, confusion, vivid dreams, excessive worry, obsessive thinking, and catastrophizing.

**Feelings.** They may experience unrealistic or excessive fear and worry about past and future events, irritability, impatience, anger, nervousness, or feeling wound up and on edge.

**Behaviors.** Anxiety can cause avoidance, obsessive or compulsive behavior, distress in social situations, sleep disturbances, and/or increased use of alcohol or drugs.

**Physical effects.** The connection between mental and physical health is fascinating. When someone is going through a mental well-being decline, as mentioned above, it can show up in their physical body, such as the physical symptoms of a panic attack, which eerily mimic a heart attack or asthma episode. (See Panic Attacks later in this chapter.)

*Anxiety Disorders*

People with anxiety problems may be diagnosed with different types of anxiety disorders. According to *Merck Manuals*, "Anxiety disorders are differentiated from one another based on the specific objects or situations that induce the fear, anxiety, and associated behavioral changes."[2] The main disorders with anxiety as a major feature are post-traumatic stress disorder, social anxiety disorder (social phobia), agoraphobia, generalized anxiety disorder, panic disorder, and obsessive-compulsive disorder. It isn't unusual for people to have more than one of these.

*Bipolar Disorder*

The Mood Disorders Society of Canada suggests: "We can all get excited by new ideas, pursue our goals with passion, and have times when we want to celebrate with our friends and enjoy life to its fullest. Conversely,

---

2. John W. Barnhill, MD, "Overview of Anxiety Disorders," *Merck Manuals*, last reviewed January 2024, accessed February 2, 2025, https://www.merckmanuals.com/professional/psychiatric-disorders/anxiety-and-stressor-related-disorders/overview-of-anxiety-disorders.

there will also be times when we're sad and withdraw into quiet contemplation or feel upset when life isn't working out as planned. For people with bipolar disorder, however, these normal emotions can become a rollercoaster ride of wild highs and devastating lows. Their moods are driven not by the events of life, but by a force of their own. Bipolar disorder (previously called manic-depressive illness) is a medical condition that involves changes in brain function leading to dramatic mood swings. These mood swings can be so severe that they impair normal functioning at work, at school, and in relationships."[3]

At times, people with bipolar disorder can experience periods of depression or mania with long periods of normal mood in between, although they usually have more episodes of depression than mania. While it's normal for our mood to change throughout the day, mood changes caused by bipolar episodes don't tend to change quickly. These episodes can last several days or even weeks.

In order for a person to be diagnosed as bipolar, there needs to be evidence of an episode of mania. It can be a challenge, however, to determine if someone has depressive disorder or bipolar disorder, as the time between episodes of depression and mania can be months apart.

The depression experienced by a person with bipolar disorder includes some or all of the symptoms of depression listed in this chapter. Mania may show up as making grand and unattainable plans or as reckless and risk-taking behavior, such as drug and alcohol misuse and having unsafe or unprotected sex. Some may feel like they're unusually important, talented, or powerful. They might spend too much money and get into debt, become angry and agitated, or get into legal trouble. In the most severe manic episodes, there's a potential for psychosis with hallucinations and delusions. The person might be very talkative, full of ideas, and have less need for sleep. Although some of these symptoms can sound beneficial (increased energy and full of ideas), mania often gets people into difficult situations.

---

3. Mood Disorders Society of Canada, "What Is Bipolar Disorder?", accessed February 2, 2025, https://mdsc.ca/edu/what-is-bipolar-disorder.

## Borderline Personality Disorder (BPD)

As described by the National Institute of Mental Health, this disorder is "a mental illness that severely impacts a person's ability to manage their emotions. This loss of emotional control can increase impulsivity, affect how they feel about themselves, and negatively impact their relationships with others. Effective treatments are available."[4]

*Signs and Symptoms of Borderline Personality Disorder*
- "Intense mood swings
- Rapid changes in how they feel about others, swinging from extreme closeness to extreme dislike and leading to unstable relationships and emotional pain
- The tendency to view things in extremes, such as all good or all bad
- Rapid changes in interests and values
- Efforts to avoid real or perceived abandonment, such as plunging headfirst into relationships or ending them just as quickly
- A pattern of intense and unstable relationships with family, friends, and loved ones
- A distorted and unstable self-image or sense of self
- Impulsive and often dangerous behaviors, such as spending sprees, unsafe sex, substance misuse, reckless driving, and binge eating
- Self-harming behavior, such as cutting
- Recurring thoughts of suicide or threats of suicide
- Intense and highly variable moods, with episodes lasting from a few hours to a few days
- Chronic feelings of emptiness
- Inappropriate, intense anger or problems controlling anger

---

4. National Institute of Mental Health, "Borderline Personality Disorder," last reviewed February 2025, accessed February 2, 2025, https://www.nimh.nih.gov/health/topics/borderline-personality-disorder.

- Feelings of dissociation, such as feeling cut off from themselves, observing themselves from outside of their body, or feelings of unreality"[5]

Not everyone with borderline personality disorder will experience all of these symptoms. The severity, frequency, and duration depend on the person and their illness. Unfortunately, borderline personality disorder can cause people to be more likely to self-harm or attempt suicide.

Sometimes, a mood disorder can be mistaken for borderline personality disorder, especially if elevated mood/energy is associated with behaviors that are reckless or impulsive.

### *Depression*

Depression is the most common mental disorder. The word *depression* is used in different ways. For many people with depression, symptoms are usually severe enough to cause noticeable problems in day-to-day activities, such as work, school, social activities, or relationships with others. Some people may feel generally miserable, unhappy, or "blue" without knowing why. Yes, we can feel sad or blue when challenging things happen, but this doesn't necessarily mean the person has a depressive disorder.

I think of the character Blue from the movie *Inside Out*, who represents the emotion of sadness and can often be seen crying. Blue doesn't hold back and naturally lets the tears flow. She uses crying as a way to slow down, release, process, and express herself, which in turn helps herself move through difficult emotions. In fact, it's proven that when people cry, they release what we call "feel good" chemicals that assist with both physical and emotional pain.

People with the "blues" or "feeling down" may have a short-term depressed mood, but with support tools and actions, they can cope and soon recover without treatment. The depression I'm referring to here is a major depressive disorder, which lasts for at least two weeks and affects a person's ability to work, carry out usual daily activities, and

---

5. Mayo Clinic Staff, "Borderline Personality Disorder," January 31, 2024, accessed February 2, 2025, https://www.mayoclinic.org/diseases-conditions/borderline-personality-disorder/symptoms-causes/syc-20370237.

have healthy personal relationships. (Bipolar disorder [discussed above] can also feature depression.)

I was floored when I learned that depression impacts approximately three hundred million people. This is a reported number. I imagine it's higher when the unreported are added. Women are nearly twice as likely to suffer from major depression than men. It's also common for depression to occur with other disorders such as substance use disorder. This is because some may look to a substance to help them with their depression symptoms.

*Signs and Symptoms of Major Depressive Disorder*
According to the Mayo Clinic, "depression may occur only once during your life, but people typically have multiple episodes. During these episodes, symptoms occur most of the day nearly every day and may include:

- Feelings of sadness, tearfulness, emptiness, or hopelessness
- Angry outbursts, irritability, or frustration, even over small matters
- Loss of interest or pleasure in most or all normal activities, such as sex, hobbies or sports
- Sleep disturbances, including insomnia or sleeping too much
- Tiredness and lack of energy, so even small tasks take extra effort
- Reduced appetite and weight loss or increased cravings for food and weight gain
- Anxiety, agitation or restlessness
- Slowed thinking, speaking or body movements
- Feelings of worthlessness or guilt, fixating on past failures or self-blame
- Trouble thinking, concentrating, making decisions and remembering things
- Frequent or recurrent thoughts of death, suicidal thoughts, suicide attempts or suicide
- Unexplained physical problems, such as back pain or headaches"[6]

---

6. Mayo Clinic Staff, "Depression (major depressive disorder)," accessed January 29, 2025, https://www.mayoclinic.org/diseases-conditions/depression/symptoms-causes/syc-20356007.

Note that not every person who is experiencing depression has all of these symptoms. People differ in the number and severity of symptoms. Even if someone doesn't have enough symptoms for a depressive disorder diagnosis, the impact on their life can still be significant. These symptoms will cause them distress and will interfere with their work and their relationships with family and friends.

While you can't diagnose depression as a layperson, you might be able to recognize the cluster of symptoms that indicate depression may be the problem. These symptoms will affect the person's thinking, feeling, behaviors, and physical well-being. Some examples include:

**Thinking.** People living with depression often have a doom and gloom vibe. Perhaps they put themselves down, or they view the world and the future through a negative lens. Their thoughts may include frequent self-criticism, self-blame, worry, pessimism, hopelessness, and helplessness. They can suffer from impaired memory and concentration, indecisiveness, confusion, a tendency to believe others see them in a negative light, and thoughts of death and suicide.

People who are depressed may say things like:

- *I'm a failure.*
- *People would be better off without me.*
- *I have let everyone down.*
- *It's all my fault.*
- *Nothing good ever happens to me.*
- *I'm worthless. I'm not worthy.*
- *No one loves me.*
- *I'm so alone.*
- *Life isn't worth living.*
- *Things will always be bad.*
- *I feel empty.*

**Feelings/Behaviors.** Depression can also involve other changes in mood or behaviors that include:

- Increased anger or irritability
- Feeling restless or on edge
- Becoming withdrawn, negative, or detached
- Increased engagement in high-risk activities
- Greater impulsivity
- Increased use and misuse of alcohol or drugs
- Isolating from family and friends
- Inability to meet the responsibilities of work and family or ignoring other important roles
- Problems with sexual desire and performance
- Sadness, anxiety, guilt, mood swings, lack of emotional responsiveness
- Crying spells
- Avoidance of social events
- Loss of interest in personal appearance, loss of motivation, slowing down, non-suicidal self-injury, sleeping too much or too little

The National Institute of Mental Health recognizes that although people of all genders can feel depressed, how they express those symptoms and the behaviors they use to cope with them may differ. For example, men may be more likely to show symptoms other than sadness, instead seeming angry or irritable. And although increased use of alcohol or drugs can be a sign of depression in anyone, men are more likely to use these substances as a coping mechanism.[7]

**Physical effects.** A range of physical symptoms are associated with depression: chronic fatigue, lack of energy, loss of appetite, constipation, weight loss or gain, headaches, irregular menstrual cycle, loss of sexual desire, and unexplained aches and pains.

A person who is depressed may be slow in moving and thinking, although they might become easily agitated. Many individuals' speech is

---

7. National Institute of Mental Health, "Depression," last reviewed January 2025, accessed January 29, 2025, https://www.nimh.nih.gov/health/topics/depression.

affected in terms of a decreased talking rate, reduced volume, and variation in tone. This is also referred to as slow, soft, and monotone speech. They may be lacking in the grooming department, too, with low interest and attention to personal hygiene and cleanliness.

They usually have a sad and depressed look, and they're often anxious, irritable, and on the verge of tears. Sometimes, depression may be harder to detect and not so obvious. Severe depression can cause the person to be emotionally unresponsive and describe themselves as "beyond tears" or emotionless.

### *Generalized Anxiety Disorder (GAD)*

Anxiety Canada describes generalized anxiety disorder (GAD) as individuals who "worry excessively and uncontrollably about daily life events and activities."[8] I refer to this as the downward spiral, or thinking of worst-case scenario(s). They often experience "uncomfortable physical symptoms, including fatigue and sore muscles, and they can also have trouble sleeping and concentrating."[9]

*Signs and Symptoms of GAD*
- Muscle tension
- Feeling keyed up or on edge
- Restlessness, irritability
- Sleep disturbance
- Avoiding news, newspapers
- Restricting involvement in activities due to excessive worries about what could happen
- Excessive seeking of reassurance or over-preparing

### *Panic Attacks*

A panic attack is a sudden episode of intense fear that triggers severe reactions when there is no real danger or apparent cause. Panic attacks

---

8. Anxiety Canada, "Generalized Anxiety Disorder in Adults," accessed January 29, 2025, https://www.anxietycanada.com/disorders/generalized-anxiety-disorder-in-adults.
9. Ibid.

are typically unexpected, coming on without any warning, and can last anywhere from a few seconds to several minutes. Although panic attacks are not life-threatening, it can be terrifying for those who experience them. In some cases, the overwhelming fear can be so intense that the individual might think they're suffering from a heart attack or other health condition.

As I write this, I'm brought back to a memory of my own experience of a panic attack. A few years back, a girlfriend gave me tickets for us to attend an outdoor SARS benefit concert with approximately five hundred thousand people in attendance. We arrived, found a spot to hang out in the general seating area, and listened to some of the bands. It was quite a lineup, including the Rolling Stones! All was well, until partway through the concert, I became overcome with fear. I felt like something really bad was going to happen. I got emotional, started to breathe heavily, and had the overwhelming feeling that I had to get out of there right away! My friend was extremely supportive. She didn't put any pressure on me to stay and helped me locate the nearest exit. The panic didn't care that I was leaving my friend behind on her own. At the time, I didn't understand what was happening. I just felt like I was losing my mind. Knowing what I do now, when these feelings start to come up, I recognize them and get support before the symptoms escalate.

Many people have a panic attack at some point in their lives. Few go on to have repeated attacks, and fewer still go on to develop panic disorder or agoraphobia. Although anyone can have a panic attack, people with anxiety disorders are more prone to them. (See Panic Disorder later in this chapter.)

*Signs and Symptoms of a Panic Attack*
A panic attack is a distinct episode of high anxiety with fear or discomfort that develops abruptly and has its peak within 10 minutes. During the attack, several of the following symptoms are usually present:

- Accelerated heart rate
- Feeling out of control
- Fear of having a heart attack

- Fear of possibly dying
- Perspiration
- Trembling hands
- Shaking throughout the body
- Tightness in the throat
- Severe shortness of breath
- Dryness in mouth
- Chills
- Sweating or hot flashes
- Upset stomach
- Abdominal cramps
- Pain or tightness in the chest
- Headache
- Dizziness or feeling lightheaded, faint, or unsteady
- Numbness or tingling sensation
- Feelings of disconnection from reality
- Feelings of exhaustion afterward
- Heart palpitations, pounding heart, or rapid heart rate
- Sensations of choking or smothering

*Panic Disorder*

As mentioned earlier, some people have short periods of extreme anxiety that's called a panic attack. It's important, however, to distinguish between a panic attack and a panic disorder. Having a panic attack doesn't necessarily mean that a person has or will develop panic disorder.

Researchers have found that several parts of the brain and certain biological processes may play a crucial role in fear and anxiety. Some researchers think panic attacks are like "false alarms" where our body's typical survival instincts are active either too often, too strongly, or some combination of the two. Researchers are studying how the brain and body interact in people with panic disorder to create more specialized treatments. In addition, they're looking at the ways stress and environmental factors play a role in the disorder.[10]

A person with panic disorder experiences recurring panic attacks and persistent worry about possible future panic attacks and their consequences for at least one month, such as a fear of losing control or having a heart attack. Some people may develop panic disorder after only a few panic attacks, while others may experience many panic attacks without developing the disorder. Others with panic disorder also develop agoraphobia (see the section on Agoraphobia earlier in this chapter), where they avoid places that they fear may cause a panic attack.

## *Phobias*

A person with a specific phobia avoids or restricts activities because of their strong fear of specific places, events, or objects. It's an intense, irrational fear of something that poses little or no actual danger. Although adults with phobias may realize that these fears are irrational, even thinking about facing the feared object or situation brings on severe anxiety symptoms. The fear is persistent, excessive, and unreasonable. Specific phobias are common but less disabling than other anxiety disorders. It's common to have some features of several of these disorders.

The most common fears are spiders, insects, mice, snakes, and heights. Other feared objects or situations might include an animal, blood, injections, storms, driving, flying, or enclosed places.

## *Post-Traumatic Stress Disorder (PTSD)*

The American Psychiatric Association describes PTSD as "a psychiatric disorder that may occur in people who have experienced or witnessed a traumatic event, series of events or set of circumstances. An individual may experience this as emotionally or physically harmful or life-threatening and may affect mental, physical, social, and/or spiritual well-being. Contrary to some misbeliefs that PTSD is something experienced through war/combat, it also includes natural disasters, severe

---

10. National Institute of Mental Health, "Panic Disorder: When Fear Overwhelms," accessed January 29, 2025, https://www.nimh.nih.gov/health/publications/panic-disorder-when-fear-overwhelms.

weather, serious accidents, terrorist acts, rape/sexual assault, historical trauma, intimate partner violence and bullying."[11] PTSD can also occur after a person is exposed to actual or threatened death, serious injury, or sexual violation.

It's common for people to feel extreme distress immediately following a traumatic event. However, if their distress lasts longer than a month, they might have PTSD. Not everyone will go on to develop a mental illness such as PTSD or depression after a traumatic event.

A common misconception is that a person must experience trauma directly to be affected. They might witness it happening to someone else, might have learned about a traumatic event occurring to someone close to them, or might have been exposed to repeated or extreme details of the event. My partner, Dave, received an unsolicited video from a friend with footage of an active shooter. He wasn't prepared and felt the effects of this video for days afterward. With access to so many of these types of videos on the internet, it's vital to recognize that witnessing traumatic situations, even though we aren't directly involved, still has an impact.

Sometimes, the memories of a traumatic event will suddenly or unexpectedly return weeks, months, or even years afterward. People can also differ a lot in how they react to these events. Particular types of traumas may affect some individuals more than others. A history of trauma may make some people more susceptible to later traumas, while others become more resilient as a result. A person who has experienced a traumatic event may react strongly right away, showing that they need immediate assistance, while others may have a delayed reaction.

*Signs and Symptoms of PTSD*
- Flashbacks
- Sleep disturbances
- Intrusive memories

---

11. American Psychiatric Foundation, "What Is Posttraumatic Stress Disorder (PTSD)?" *Psychiatry.org*, reviewed November 2022, accessed January 29, 2025, https://www.psychiatry.org/patients-families/ptsd/what-is-ptsd.

- Persistently negative thoughts
- Low mood, anger, or feeling emotionally numb
- Triggers, such as sounds, sights, smells, thoughts, or memories that remind them of the traumatic event
- Trouble feeling emotionally connected to family or close friends
- Remembering the event often and vividly
- Trouble remembering parts of the event (amnesia) or trying to avoid remembering it

*Psychosis*

This is a general term to describe a mental health problem in which a person has lost some contact with reality. According to the Yale School of Medicine, "a person who is going through an episode of psychosis can experience an alteration in their perceptions of reality and can have difficulty thinking clearly as they normally would. When someone is affected in this way, they may have unusual or strange ideas, they may hear or see things that aren't there, and they may have problems managing their emotions. Psychosis is most likely to occur in young adults and is quite common. About three out of every one hundred young people will experience a psychotic episode. Most make a full recovery from the experience. But psychosis can happen to anyone. An episode of psychosis is treatable, and it's possible to recover. It's widely accepted that the earlier people get help, the better the outcome. Twenty-five percent of people who develop psychosis will never have another episode. Another 50 percent may have more than one episode but will be able to live normal lives. Some people who develop psychosis may need ongoing support and treatment throughout their lives."[12]

There are numerous disorders in which a person can experience psychosis, including schizophrenia, psychotic depression, bipolar disorder (which can involve psychotic depression or psychotic mania), schizoaffective disorder, and drug-induced psychosis.

---

12. Yale School of Medicine, "What Is Psychosis?", accessed January 29, 2025, https://medicine.yale.edu/psychiatry/step/psychosis.

People usually experience psychosis in episodes:

- **Acute (psychotic phase)**—the person is unwell with psychotic symptoms such as delusions, hallucinations, disorganized thinking, and reduction in the ability to work, study, or maintain social relationships.
- **Recovery**—an individual process the person goes through to attain a level of well-being.
- **Relapse**—the person may only have one episode in their life or may go on to have relapse episodes.

*Psychotic Depression.* Sometimes, depression can be so intense that it causes psychotic symptoms. A person with psychotic depression will also usually experience delusions, hallucinations, and voices, beliefs that they're inadequate, guilt about something that wasn't their fault, beliefs that they're being persecuted or observed, or become severely physically ill.

*Bipolar Disorder with Psychosis.* Sometimes, a person with bipolar disorder may also experience delusions and hallucinations, which is called psychotic mania. This involves grandiose beliefs about their abilities or invulnerability. They may not be aware that they're in mania, they might feel their delusions are real, and they may not be aware they're ill.

*Substance-Induced Psychosis.* According to the National Drug and Alcohol Research Centre, "substance-induced psychosis is a form of psychosis brought on by alcohol or other drug use. It can also occur when a person is withdrawing from alcohol or other drugs. The most common symptoms include visual hallucinations, disorientation, and memory problems.

Symptoms usually appear quickly and resolve within days to weeks. However, the person may have another psychotic episode in the future if they use that drug again. While substance-induced psychosis is typically brief, alcohol or other drug use can trigger the onset of longer-lasting psychotic disorders in individuals who are predisposed to developing them."[13]

---

13. K. Mills et al., *Psychosis + Substance Use*, National Drug and Alcohol Research Centre, 2011, accessed February 2, 2025, https://ndarc.med.unsw.edu.au/sites/default/files/ndarc/resources/NDARC_PYCHOSIS_FINAL.pdf.

## How Do You Recognize the Signs/Symptoms of Mental Health Decline?

*Signs and Symptoms When Psychosis Is Developing*
- Suspiciousness, paranoid ideas, or uneasiness with others
- Depression, anxiety, irritability
- Trouble thinking clearly and logically
- Withdrawing socially and spending a lot more time alone
- Difficulties with concentration or attention; a sense of alteration of self, others, or the outside world (feeling that self or others have changed or are acting differently in some way)
- Unusual or overly intense ideas, strange feelings, or a lack of feeling
- Different perceptual experiences (a reduction or greater intensity of smell, sound, or color)
- Decline in self-care or personal hygiene
- Disruption of sleep, including difficulty falling asleep and reduced sleep time
- Difficulty telling reality from fantasy
- Confused speech or trouble communicating
- Sudden drop in grades or job performance

Not everyone will experience the same signs and symptoms, and they can change over time. An individual symptom may be difficult enough to manage on its own, but when symptoms happen together, it's a good indication something isn't right. It's important not to ignore or dismiss such warning signs and symptoms, even if they appear gradually and are unclear. Don't assume that the person is just going through a phase or that the symptoms will go away on their own.

Note that depending on the spiritual and cultural context of the person's behaviors, the interpretation of a symptom of psychosis in one culture may be perceived as normal in another culture.

### *Schizophrenia*
Psychosis is most common in schizophrenia. Contrary to common belief, this mental illness is not a "split personality." The term *schizophrenia*

comes from the Greek word for "fractured mind" and refers to changes in mental function where thoughts and perceptions become disordered.

The Cleveland Clinic defines schizophrenia as a "psychiatric condition that has severe effects on your physical and mental well-being. It disrupts how your brain works, interfering with things like your thoughts, memory, senses and behaviors. As a result, you may struggle in many parts of your day-to-day life. Untreated schizophrenia often disrupts your relationships (professional, social, romantic and otherwise). It can also cause you to have trouble organizing your thoughts, and you might behave in ways that put you at risk for injuries or other illnesses."[14]

*Signs and Symptoms of Schizophrenia*
Per the *DSM-5* Criteria for Schizophrenia, two (or more) of the following must each present for a significant portion of time during a one-month period (or less if successfully treated) for a diagnosis of schizophrenia. At least one of these must be (1), (2), or (3):

1. *Delusions.* False beliefs even if evidence is given to the contrary.

2. *Hallucinations.* Can see, smell, feel, hear things that don't exist. For example, hearing voices.

3. *Disorganized speech.* When speaking, challenged with organizing thoughts. They might jump all over the place. I describe this as a "word salad." Changing topics frequently and difficulty staying on topic.

4. *Catatonic behavior.* Affects movement, speech, and behaviors in several different ways. They may be awake, but they don't seem to respond to other people or their environment.

5. *Negative symptoms.* Loss of ability to do things as usual. Their voice might change or become flat and emotionless.

---

14. Cleveland Clinic, "Schizophrenia," last reviewed December 11, 2024, accessed February 2, 2025, https://my.clevelandclinic.org/health/diseases/4568-schizophrenia.

### *Social Anxiety Disorder (Social Phobia)*

The Centre for Addictions and Mental Health refers to this disorder as "involving a fear or anxiety about being humiliated or scrutinized in social situations, which lasts at least six months. This fear causes significant distress or impairment in day-to-day functioning (e.g., social or occupational). Fears may be associated with social interactions, being observed and/or performing. Examples include meeting strangers, dating, participating in small groups or playing sports."[15] The key fear is that others will think badly of them.

For example, I previously mentioned a client whose wife refused to go to functions with friends or family, as she was consumed with social anxiety, low self-esteem, and low self-worth. She was riddled with thoughts like "I've put on so much weight" and "I'm so embarrassed." Nothing he tried helped her get over the fear so that she could attend the events.

### *Substance Use Problems*

Contrary to the stigma, using a substance doesn't mean a person will have substance use problems. They occur when the person uses alcohol and/or drugs at levels that are associated with short-term or long-term harm. It isn't just a matter of how much a person uses, but how their use affects their life and those around them. To have a substance use disorder, their problems must have an adverse effect on their life during the past year in two or more of the following areas, the most common as listed here by Johns Hopkins Medicine:

*Symptoms may include:*

- Using or drinking larger amounts or over longer periods of time than planned.
- Continually wanting or unsuccessfully trying to cut down or control use of drugs or alcohol.
- Spending a lot of time getting, using, or recovering from use of drugs or alcohol.

---

15. CAMH, "Social Anxiety Disorder," accessed January 29, 2025, https://www.camh.ca/en/health-info/mental-illness-and-addiction-index/social-anxiety-disorder.

- Craving, or a strong desire to use drugs or alcohol.
- Ongoing drug or alcohol use that interferes with work, school, or home duties.
- Using drugs or alcohol even with continued relationship problems caused by use.
- Giving up or reducing activities because of drug or alcohol use.
- Taking risks, such as sexual risks or driving under the influence.
- Continually using drugs or alcohol even though it is causing or adding to physical or psychological problems.
- Developing tolerance or the need to use more drugs or alcohol to get the same effect. Or using the same amount of drugs or alcohol, but without the same effect.
- Having withdrawal symptoms if not using drugs or alcohol. Or using alcohol or another drug to avoid such symptoms.[16]

Substance use disorders often co-occur with other mental health disorders such as anxiety disorders, depression, attention-deficit hyperactivity disorder (ADHD), bipolar disorder, personality disorders, and schizophrenia. Alcohol or other drugs can also cause additional problems in someone's life with finances or in relationships, for example, and heavy use may contribute to or exacerbate a mental illness. Please note that even though someone might have both a substance use disorder and another mental disorder, it doesn't necessarily mean that one caused the other.

*Alcohol Use Problems*
Alcohol makes people less alert and impairs concentration and coordination. Some people use it to reduce anxiety, so in the short term, it can be helpful in this regard. In small quantities, alcohol causes people to relax

---

16. Johns Hopkins Medicine, "Substance Use Disorder," accessed February 2, 2025, https://www.hopkinsmedicine.org/health/conditions-and-diseases/substance-abuse-chemical-dependency.

and lower their inhibitions. They can feel more confident, so people often become more extroverted when using it.

However, alcohol use can produce a range of short-term and long-term problems. This research-based information on drinking and its impact comes from the National Institute on Alcohol Abuse and Alcoholism:

*Drinking too much* on a single occasion or over time can take a serious toll on your health. Here's how alcohol can affect your body:

*Brain:* Alcohol interferes with the brain's communication pathways, and can affect the way the brain looks and works. These disruptions can change mood and behavior, and make it harder to think clearly and move with coordination.

*Heart:* Drinking a lot over a long time or too much on a single occasion can damage the heart, causing problems including:

Cardiomyopathy—Stretching and drooping of heart muscle

Arrhythmias—Irregular heartbeat

Stroke

High blood pressure

*Liver:* Heavy drinking takes a toll on the liver, and can lead to a variety of problems and liver inflammations including:

- Steatosis or fatty liver
- Alcoholic hepatitis
- Fibrosis
- Cirrhosis

*Pancreas:* Alcohol causes the pancreas to produce toxic substances that can eventually lead to pancreatitis, a dangerous inflammation in the pancreas that causes its swelling and pain (which may spread) and impairs its ability to make enzymes and hormones for proper digestion.[17]

---

17. National Institute of Alcohol Abuse and Alcoholism, "Alcohol's Effects on the Body," last reviewed June 6, 2024, accessed February 2, 2025, https://www.niaaa.nih.gov/alcohols-effects-health/alcohols-effects-body.

As well as causing serious health problems, long-term alcohol misuse can lead to social problems for some people, such as unemployment, divorce, domestic abuse, sexual abuse, homelessness, suicide, and self-injury.

*Drug Use Problems*

There is a wide variety of other drugs that can cause problems and lead to substance use disorders.

*Cannabis (marijuana)* is a mind-altering drug that is a mixture of dried, shredded leaves, stems, seeds, and flowers of the hemp plant. The main active chemical in cannabis is THC (delta-9-tetrahydrocannabinol). The effects of cannabis vary depending on how much THC a cannabis product contains. The THC content of cannabis has been increasing since the 1970s.

The Center for Disease Control and Prevention states that

*cannabis use can cause disorientation and sometimes unpleasant thoughts or feelings of anxiety and paranoia.*

*People who use cannabis are more likely to develop long-lasting mental disorders, including schizophrenia. The association between cannabis and schizophrenia is stronger in people who start using cannabis at an earlier age and use cannabis more frequently.*

*Cannabis use is also associated with depression; social anxiety; and thoughts of suicide, suicide attempts, and suicide.*[18]

*Opioids* "are a class of natural, semi-synthetic, and synthetic drugs that include both prescription medications and illegal drugs like heroin. Prescription medications such as oxycodone (OxyContin), hydrocodone (Vicodin), morphine, codeine, fentanyl, and others are mainly used for the treatment of pain."[19] Some people will become dependent on these medications after long-term use. Older people are the most likely to be affected.

Long-term use of these medications can increase the risk of falls and cognitive impairment in older people.

---

18. https://www.cdc.gov/cannabis/health-effects/mental-health.html.
19. National Institute on Drug Abuse, "Opioids," November 2024, accessed February 2, 2025, https://nida.nih.gov/research-topics/opioids#opioids.

*Cocaine* is a highly addictive stimulant drug turned into a white powder from coca leaves. "Some nicknames include blow, coca, coke, crack, crank, flake, rock, snow, soda and cot. Cocaine is an intense, euphoria-producing stimulant drug with strong addictive potential even after using it for a very short time."[20] With long-term use, people can develop mental health and substance use problems such as paranoia, aggression, anxiety, and depression. Cocaine can also bring on an episode of drug-induced psychosis.

*Amphetamines (including methamphetamine).* "Amphetamines are generally taken orally or injected. However, the addition of 'ice,' the slang name of crystallized methamphetamine hydrochloride, has promoted smoking as another mode of administration. Just as 'crack' is smokable cocaine, 'ice' is smokable methamphetamine."[21] These drugs belong to a category of stimulants and have the temporary effect of increasing energy and apparent mental alertness. Once the effect wears off, the person may experience a range of problems, including depression, irritability, agitation, increased appetite, and sleepiness.

Amphetamines come in many shapes and forms, including powder, tablets, capsules, crystals, or liquid. Methamphetamine (meth) has a chemical structure similar to that of amphetamine, but it has stronger effects on the brain that can last for six to eight hours. After the initial "rush," the person may experience a state of agitation, which can lead to violent behavior in some individuals.

When someone goes into an amphetamine psychosis or "speed psychosis," it's a mental health risk because the person may experience symptoms similar to schizophrenia. They may have hallucinations, delusions, and uncontrolled violent behaviors, as mentioned in the section on psychosis. They will recover as the drug wears off but will be vulnerable to further episodes of drug-induced psychosis if the drug is used again.

Some types of amphetamines have legitimate medical uses under a prescription to treat ADHD and other medical conditions.

---

20. US Drug Enforcement Administration, "Cocaine," accessed February 2, 2025, https://www.dea.gov/factsheets/cocaine.
21. US Drug Enforcement Administration, "Amphetamines," accessed February 2, 2025, https://www.dea.gov/factsheets/amphetamines.

*Suicide*

The World Health Organization says that annually, more than 720,000 people worldwide commit suicide.[22] The numbers are much higher if you add those who make attempts on their life. Here are some common warning signs, according to the Suicide Prevention Resource Center:

*Talking about:*

- Feeling unbearable pain
- Death or a recent fascination with death
- Feeling hopeless, worthless, or trapped
- Feeling guilt, shame, or anger
- Feeling like they are a burden to others

*Changes in behavior or mood:*

- Recent suicide attempt
- Increased alcohol or drug use
- Losing interest in personal appearance or hygiene
- Withdrawing from family, friends, or community
- Saying goodbye to friends and family
- Giving away prized possessions
- A recent episode of depression, emotional distress, and/or anxiety
- Changes in eating and/or sleeping patterns
- Becoming violent or being a victim of violence
- Expressing rage
- Recklessness[23]

---

22. World Health Organization, "Suicide," August 29, 2024, accessed February 2, 2025, https://www.who.int/news-room/fact-sheets/detail/suicide.

23. Suicide Prevention Resource Center, "Warning Signs of Suicide," accessed February 2, 2025, https://sprc.org/warning-signs-of-suicide.

People may show one or many of these signs, and some may show signs not on this list. Always err on the side of caution if you think someone is considering suicide. Even if you only have a mild suspicion, approach them and ask if they're thinking of dying by suicide. I used to think if I asked them that, it was like a form of encouragement or planting a seed. But it isn't—it actually lets them know that someone cares enough about them to ask. Share your concerns, and describe the behaviors that have caused you to worry. Understand that the person may not want to speak with you, however. In this instance, offer to help them find someone else to talk to. Livingworks offers global informative programs such as SafeTalk and Assist. These courses go into more detail about how to support someone looking to die by suicide and how to have those conversations.

Take all thoughts of suicide seriously, and take action immediately. Never dismiss the person's thoughts as "attention-seeking." Determine the urgency of taking action based on your recognition of the suicide warning signs, and inquire about issues that affect their immediate safety. I understand it can feel awkward to call for help, but if you feel the person is at risk, do it anyway.

## Dementia

According to The Dementia Society, dementia itself isn't a disease. Instead, it describes a variety of neurological disorders that affect the brain and prevent people from functioning normally.[24]

*Signs and Symptoms of Dementia*

*Early signs and symptoms are:*

- Forgetting things or recent events
- Losing or misplacing things
- Getting lost when walking or driving

---

24. Dementia Society of America, "Definitions," accessed February 2, 2025, https://www.dementiasociety.org/definitions?gad_source=1&gclid=EAIaIQobChMIk83nnO6diwMVok7_AR3YlwTjEAAYAiAAEgI_4PD_BwE.

- Confusion, even in familiar places
- Losing track of time
- Difficulty solving problems or making decisions
- Problems following conversations or finding words
- Struggles with performing familiar tasks
- Misjudging distances to objects visually

*Common changes in mood and behavior include:*

- Feeling anxious, sad, or angry about memory loss
- Personality changes
- Inappropriate behaviors
- Withdrawal from work or social activities
- Less interest in other people's emotions
- Aggression

*Later symptoms of dementia include:*

- Difficulty recognizing family members or friends
- Difficulty moving around
- Loss of control over bladder and bowels
- Trouble eating and drinking[25]

## JUICY BITS

Our degree of mental and/or physical health can change based on many factors. Being aware of the signs and symptoms of a mental well-being decline is a great start in supporting yourself and others. In the Mental Health First Aid certification course, we share a video of managers and staff in the workforce sharing their self-stigma about having a mental health problem, illness, and/or crisis. One participant was surprised after watching the video, recognizing that she used to work with someone who

---

25. World Health Organization, "Dementia," March 15, 2023, accessed February 2, 2025, https://www.who.int/news-room/fact-sheets/detail/dementia.

appeared in it. She shared that if she had known what that person was experiencing, it would have changed the dynamic of their challenging relationship. She would have been willing to help her coworker more. So the more knowledgeable we are in recognizing these signs and symptoms, the more we have the opportunity to get support early and validate the experiences of others.

## Exercise: Journaling About Signs and Symptoms You Observe

For the purpose of our time together, I recommend getting a journal (if you don't already have one). As we go through the chapters, I'll invite you to note what stood out for you, and I'll often provide an exercise to help you apply what you learned in your own life.

1. Please make note of any signs or symptoms that you may have recognized in yourself and/or your loved ones.

2. How have these signs or symptoms impacted your life to date?

CHAPTER THREE

# The Four As: Awareness, Acknowledgment, Acceptance, and Action = Change

ONE OF THE BIGGEST "AHA!" MOMENTS I HAVE HAD TO DATE HAPPENED when I was studying to become a psychotherapist. We had to do our own personal therapy as an individual and in groups. In those groups, I recognized that others had similar feelings and experiences to mine. Once I became aware that what I was feeling and experiencing were natural responses to some of the challenges in my life, this made a world of difference. To this day, having this awareness empowers me to make different choices/actions to show up healthier in relationships, work, and my community.

The following formula has worked well in my life in many situations:

**Awareness, Acknowledgment, Acceptance, and Action = Change**

I call these the Four As.

First, we must become aware of what's happening. Chapter 2 was largely about that—recognizing the signs and symptoms of mental health decline. This awareness is key.

Acknowledgment takes awareness a step further, as we acknowledge that our situation is painful or difficult.

Acceptance then takes acknowledgment yet another step further. We don't just recognize that our situation is challenging. We stop shoving issues under the carpet and start to accept the truth of the matter. This doesn't mean that we like it or agree with it. Too often, we think if we accept something, it means we're happy with it. But no, as the Buddhists say, we accept "what is" because that's when we leave any traces of denial behind us and see our situation realistically. We make peace with what's true. Then and only then can we determine the proper action to take.

Action is the last of the Four As. When we act based on a realistic view of what's happening, we can see the benefits of true change. We might not be able to "fix" someone else's mental well-being decline, but we can make a difference, if not for them, then for ourselves.

Over the next few pages, we'll dive into some of the issues that may arise as you navigate yourself through a loved one's mental well-being decline. Each topic falls under one of the Four As.

They aren't related to any one specific disorder, problem, or crisis. If your loved one is living with bipolar disorder, substance use, anxiety, borderline personality disorder, dementia, or something else, the principles for you will still apply. They're universal.

### Awareness: Operation Night Watch

On a recent trip to Amsterdam, I was reminded of the importance of the Four As to preserve our own well-being. At the Rijks Museum there, Operation Night Watch is the largest and most wide-ranging research and conservation project in the history of Rembrandt's masterpiece, "Night Watch." Using a series of groundbreaking tools and techniques, they monitor outside factors that affect the art with the intention of providing the best environment to preserve the painting long-term with as little disruption as possible. These influences include vibrations that are created with sound and energy while the public views the work, as well as heat and air-conditioning elements. They are also researching what might be the best frame, backing, and protection for the painting.

Like Operation Night Watch, you need to become aware of the emotional factors that influence you—the masterpiece. Are you acknowledging the impact of these emotions on your own mental and physical well-being? Let's dive deep into what some of these emotional elements might be for you.

The Four As: Awareness, Acknowledgment, Acceptance, and Action = Change

## Awareness: Emotional Inflammation

When triggered by the immune system, inflammation plays a key role in the body, protecting us from infection, injury, and disease. However, when inflammation goes wrong or becomes chronic, we are more susceptible to disease. The effects of inflammation can be a good indicator that we need to pay attention.

When we become aware of it, we need to find the source. For example, eating certain foods can cause inflammation. Similarly, what are you "feeding" your mind? Just like our body, our mind can create dis-ease that's equivalent to inflammation.

The term *emotional inflammation* was recently coined by authors Lise Van Susteren, MD and Stacey Colino in their book, *Emotional Inflammation: Discover Your Triggers and Reclaim Your Equilibrium During Anxious Times*. It's caused by extreme stress and pressure, such as intense emotions, negative thoughts, an environment where we're surrounded by struggle, and/or circumstances that are too much to handle. When dealing with a loved one's mental well-being decline, you may not realize how often you're in a state of emotional inflammation.

Signs that you might be emotionally inflamed can include irritability, lethargy, consuming more food or a substance than usual, wanting to isolate, scrolling social media for hours on end, feeling unmotivated for daily activities, and feeling overemotional, to name a few.

On any given day, we can consider ourselves to be "emotionally sound," meaning that we feel calm and equipped to deal with anything that comes our way. During extremely stressful times, however, we're more susceptible to exhaustion and illness, and struggle to cope with what comes. When your emotional resources are low, you're likely experiencing emotional inflammation.

A couple shared a situation with me that occurred when the wife had a mental health crisis. She had an emotional outburst that included screaming, shouting, throwing things, and putting holes in walls. The event escalated until the police were called. When they arrived on the scene, she implied her husband was abusive to her. The officers separated them and got each of them to tell their side of the story.

The husband was exhausted and full of emotional turmoil from his wife's mental illness. Out of desperation, he begged the officer to take him away in handcuffs. Usually, he'd be able to cope with these types of outbursts, as they'd been happening many times over several years. But he became so overwhelmed with living in that environment that he could no longer handle it. He had become emotionally inflamed and needed to pay attention to his own needs.

It's imperative that we become aware of our own limitations, which means knowing what we can and can't do when a loved one is in crisis.

## Awareness: Guilt

Guilt is an unpleasant emotion that we feel when we believe we've done something wrong that hurt someone else. It isn't uncommon for people to feel guilty about their loved one's mental illness. They might falsely believe that they gave the illness to their loved one.

Sometimes, we confuse guilt with shame, but guilt is associated with something we believe we *did*, while shame is a feeling of worthlessness associated with *who we are*.

Shame is never legitimate, but guilt can be. We may have made a mistake that hurt someone and may owe them an apology. You might feel guilty, for example, for becoming irritated with your loved one's excessive neediness. Maybe you feel guilty for not being as "loyal" to your loved one as you believe you should have been.

In this book, I've shared experiences I've had with my mother, and I've had moments of feeling guilty about it, even though she always encouraged me to write a book. Am I being unloyal for sharing such personal, sensitive experiences? At times, I hear her in my ear, cheering me on, but the guilty feelings still come up. I frequently look at the picture of her on my desk and nod to her in acknowledgment.

You aren't being disloyal to the person you love when you keep yourself miserable and in pain. You might feel it keeps you connected to them, but I invite you to consider that your loved one doesn't want to see you unhappy either.

I've had several people share that they felt guilty as their life came together, while their loved one was suffering. But you have done nothing "wrong" when you succeed. Your loved one needs you to do well. When someone has it "worse" than you, it doesn't mean you don't have a right to prosper.

To alleviate feelings of guilt for what my mom was going through, I sometimes took responsibility for her moods and tried to change them. She always considered me to be her "ray of sunshine." In my codependency, I believed it was my job to make her feel good, and honestly, I was really good at it. In fact, for years, I got good at trying to change other people's moods, too! I'm still highly sensitive to the people in my environment, but now, I make a conscious effort not to feel guilty when they don't feel good, even when I do.

If you're experiencing guilt, please become aware of those feelings, and ask yourself if the guilt is truly merited. Or are you putting undue expectations on yourself or taking too much responsibility for your loved one's mental health challenges?

### AWARENESS AND ACKNOWLEDGMENT: ANGER AND RESENTMENT

Did you ever see the movie *Inside Out*? It teaches us that every emotion has a purpose. Although the characters are cartoons targeted to children, I believe it's a fabulous movie for all ages.

There's a character in it named Anger, who is very serious, temperamental, sarcastic, strict, wrathful, somewhat antagonistic, and very closed when expressing sadness or happiness.

When we try to help a loved one with a mental health issue, we might be met with anger. No matter how much we support our loved one, bend over backwards, and go out of our way, we might still be seen as the "bad guy." That, of course, is likely to make us feel angry in response.

Anger comes up when there's little to no appreciation for what we do to help. We feel it when our loved one's symptoms cause them to act out in damaging ways like putting holes in walls, slashing tires, or stealing money. Sometimes, caregivers even risk losing their job because they drop everything to help their loved one in a crisis. Anger certainly comes up when we receive countless promises that the behaviors will change, but they never do.

It's understandable to feel anger in these situations, but when left unchecked, it can turn into resentment and bitterness because we feel mistreated or wronged. We might even adopt an "us versus them" attitude that eventually causes physical and mental health issues. Maybe we feel resentful for providing for our loved one, giving them a safe place to live, food on the table, driving them everywhere, and doing whatever we can to keep them from the substance they may be abusing. Yet, their behaviors continue despite their promises to stop.

When resentment shows up, it's a sign that we need to become aware of our anger so that we can acknowledge and feel it, even if we feel guilty about it. When we deny it, we're much more likely to lash out at someone. When we acknowledge it, we can find healthy outlets for it, whether through therapy, journaling, meditation, or something else. Letting the emotions out without hurting someone else in the process can help us avoid shouting matches with our loved ones.

### Awareness and Acknowledgment: Anxiety

As we talked about in Chapter 2, anxiety can be debilitating, although it can also protect us by helping us move quickly into action when our safety is threatened. But let's discuss the anxiety that leaves us feeling nervous, depleted, and on edge when we're dealing with a loved one who's going through a mental health decline.

I think of anxiety as being stuck in the "what ifs." *What if the next time my loved one says they'll die, they do? What if they're in danger? What if they don't come home?* As my mom used to say, anxiety is "future thinking." It's important to acknowledge these "what ifs" so that we can deal with them from a more objective point of view than our anxiety. What are some of the "what ifs" you say to yourself?

Sometimes, anxiety and physical pain are difficult to distinguish from one another. When my mother was on her deathbed, she was full of anxiety about dying. She woke up periodically in a panic, remembering that she was dying of cancer. She'd say, "What can I do? What can I do?" I think she hoped we would somehow have an answer that would stop her from dying. It was awful.

Part of her palliative care regime was to manage her pain and anxiety. The medication was administered with a pump connected intravenously, which we could press periodically when there was a need, and it was set with limits to avoid an overdose.

When my mother woke up with cries of pain, it was hard to distinguish if the pain was physical or mental. I'd ask her which meds she needed. "Are you having physical pain or anxiety?" More often than not, she would tell me it was anxiety.

She was very aware of her mental health issues, even on her deathbed. Living with mental illness had blessed her with a bag full of tools to ease her symptoms. One of those tools was denial.

At one point while Mom was asleep, my dad and I discussed the news the doctor had shared with all of us earlier. She suddenly woke up and said, "Stop talking about it! I don't want to know!" It was her way of coping with the situation.

It's terrible to watch a loved one experience extreme anxiety. There was very little I could do to help her other than accept her feelings and do my best to create a space of love and peace. Sometimes, that's all we can do.

I have also personally experienced acute anxiety many times, and when others are in a state of anxiety, it triggers my own. Having this awareness has helped me recognize the tools I need to support myself, which we'll discuss later in the book.

## Acknowledgment: The Clear Out

I often include visits with friends and family when I travel to speak about mental health. I welcome the quality time, and the conversations tend to end up "on purpose." On a recent trip across Canada, a family member named Sandra, who is a veteran teacher in British Columbia, shared some of the mental health challenges that students witness.

When a student is having a decline, it can lead to a mental health crisis, and their symptoms affect the entire classroom, including the teacher. Their fellow students react in a variety of ways. Some want to make the person feel better, others feel fearful, some cry or experience anxiety, and some take on the attitude that they've seen it before. The latter students tend to guide the other students to let the one in crisis "just be." They have an *awareness* that they can't "fix" it.

This reminded me of how we all react in varying ways when we're on the receiving end of someone's symptoms (lashing out, hurtful words, or strong emotions). So I invite you to reflect on how you respond/react when met with a loved one's mental well-being symptoms. Do you *acknowledge* how you feel? What *action* do you take?

*Acknowledging* how the child in crisis impacts others, teachers often go into *action* and do what they refer to as a "room clear." This action comes from a "ready to go tub" that Sandra prepares, which contains a couple of activities kids can do in an alternate environment inside or outside the class. The activities include crosswords, math and science work, and drawing prompts to be done indoors. Outdoor activities include scavenger hunts, bug hunts, tree identifications, and nature art or math.

The goal is to remove students from the room where they would witness the child who is in crisis, both for the dignity of that child and to support the mental health of the other kids. This has proven to be one of the better ways to provide a psychological safe space for all involved.

### Acknowledgment: The Emotional Rock Garden

My front garden has a variety of rocks spread out between the plants as part of the design. I noticed over the years that the rocks were disappearing, so I asked my good friend, Lisa, who helped with the planting, where I could get more rocks. She laughed and said, "They aren't disappearing, Yvette. They've just sunken further into the ground." She suggested I dig up the partially covered rocks and bring them back to the surface. It got me thinking about how we do that in life. Rather than seeing what's already there, we add more or cover up to avoid feeling our emotions. We numb and distract ourselves.

But when we push down our uncomfortable emotions, we also push down our joy, happiness, faith, hope, and more. Acknowledging our emotions and pain is a form of planting seeds for future growth. Part of our healing requires digging and allowing our feelings to surface. Once we hear and feel them, we can witness their beauty just like the rocks I unearthed from my garden.

What's your emotional rock garden look like? I invite you to tend to your emotions by digging deep and planting seeds for healing and growth.

## ACKNOWLEDGMENT: DON'T BITE THE HAND THAT FEEDS YOU

As a child, I bit my nails. This was explained away as a "bad habit." I tried special nail polish with a bitter taste, but I still sometimes gnawed away at my nails and cuticles until I drew blood. This "habit" lasted well into my adulthood.

Eventually, someone pointed out that when I bite myself, I'm not just biting my nails. I'm biting myself! I was attacking me! It was like biting the hand that feeds you.

Acknowledging this was a game-changer. As a result, I started to pay attention to when I started to bite my nails and asked myself what was "eating away" at me. What was causing me to harm myself? The answer wasn't always the same, but that awareness and acknowledgment were key.

Today, I don't bite myself. I'm aware that when I start to play with my nails, it's a clue that something is causing me stress. I then go inward to tap into how I'm feeling.

Those of us who care for a loved one in mental health decline often end up biting the hand that feeds us because we tend to put our own needs on the back burner and avoid taking care of ourselves. But when we ignore our emotions, they show up in other areas. This is what happened with my nail-biting. That behavior was a manifestation of ignoring my emotions and needs. No matter how much your loved one may need you, it's vital that you also take care of yourself.

## ACKNOWLEDGMENT: POLLYANNA-ISH

Some of you may be familiar with the 1913 novel, *Pollyanna*, by American author Eleanor H. Porter, which is considered a classic of children's literature. The character of Pollyanna, also known as the "Glad Girl," had irrepressible optimism even in the face of the most adverse circumstances. In modern day slang, the Pollyanna principle is used to describe our tendency to remember pleasant memories more accurately than unpleasant ones. Research indicates that at the subconscious level, our minds tend to focus on optimism, while at the conscious level, it tends to focus on the negative.

I have been called "Pollyanna" many times in my life. I tend to be the silver lining, chin up, the show must go on, everything happens for a reason, nothing a "good cuppa" couldn't solve (referencing my British/Irish heritage) kind of gal. In the past, it was common for me to put on a brave face for others, smiling even when I had no desire to smile.

But acknowledging the truth of our circumstances is the start of change. For a long time, I bypassed what I was truly feeling. A short time after my mom died, I was on a weekend getaway with one of my best friends and her mother, MK. In hindsight, it may have been too soon for me to be social. I carried on in my usual smiley way, not wanting to put a damper on anyone's good time. But MK has volunteered in hospice care for years, bringing comfort to those who are dying and to the loved ones who are grieving. At the end of the trip, we had a quiet moment together, and she reminded me that I don't have to always smile or be upbeat and joyful. She reminded me not to bypass my feelings, to get in touch with them, to speak them aloud, and to let them out. I will always remember that moment.

I teach this, too, now, but I still needed the reminder. We can't "put lipstick on a pig," as the phrase goes, which means trying to hide the truth. So I recommend acknowledging your situation for what it is, not what you'd like it to be.

When a loved one is ill, physically or mentally, it sucks! It hurts, and it's discouraging, frustrating, exhausting, maddening, and scarring. I invite you to add your own descriptive words to the list and acknowledge them all.

## Acknowledgment: Emotions Need Motion

Can you relate to any of the following?

- Being afraid to upset the other person
- Feeling you've lost your sense of self—who you are

## The Four As: Awareness, Acknowledgment, Acceptance, and Action = Change

- Constantly checking your thoughts before you speak
- Being in a constant state of tension and anxiety
- Always second-guessing yourself
- Always assuming you did something wrong

Psychology once assumed that most human emotions fall within the universal categories of happiness, sadness, anger, surprise, fear, and disgust. A new study identifies twenty-seven categories of emotion and shows how they blend together in our everyday experiences. Yet, most of us were never taught how to describe or name our feelings.

Brené Brown hosts an informative, human-centered TV series called *Atlas of the Heart* (and wrote a book with the same title) that dives deep into defining emotions and the words used to describe them.

Let's acknowledge how *you* feel in response to symptoms you observe in a loved one. After all, emotions need motion. It's important to stop pushing them down, name them, feel them, and release them.

Don't judge the reason for your tears. They could be brought on by a movie, commercial, hurt feelings, happiness, physical pain, grief, fear, connection with someone else, and many more reasons. I invite you to stop and reflect on what brings on the waterworks for you.

There is still so much self-stigma in our society about tears, and there are many misconceptions from others about what's happening when someone cries. But crying can result from temporary sadness or feeling moved. It doesn't mean someone is necessarily depressed. We all have sadness at times in our life. So give yourself permission to have a good old fashioned snot cry or "ugly cry." This is the kind where you wake up in the morning with red, swollen eyes and stuffy sinuses. Although you may experience some physical unpleasantness, it's temporary, and your mental health will thank you for it.

### Acknowledgment: Numbing Out

The ability to feel emotions allows us to live a more fulfilling life. So what happens when our emotions prove to be too much? Sometimes, the brain's solution is to shut our feelings off altogether, creating emotional numbness, which is sometimes called emotional apathy. This is a normal response to intense stress.

Our brain does a great job of assessing situations and finding ways to increase our feeling of safety. So emotional numbing can be beneficial temporarily, but it isn't an effective long-term coping strategy.

How do you know if you're emotionally numbing? You may feel like you're invisible, separated from everyone else. The world around you may not feel real, and you might feel like you're watching life from a distance like a movie. You may have a lingering sense of emptiness, like something is missing, and you can't focus or engage with what's happening around you.

Emotional numbing can restrict your ability to experience happiness or joy, even toward those who have been a source of joy for you in the past. So it's vital to become aware of this and acknowledge it. You might need therapy in order to move yourself out of this state, especially if you've been numb for a long time. You may feel stuck in it. So get the help you need to get unstuck because you owe it to yourself to have a life that's filled with joy, even if it means you have to sometimes also feel pain. It really is worth it!

## Acknowledgment: Ground Control to Major Tom

One of my best friends, Kim, lost a parent to a substance use disorder. She told me that the most challenging emotion she felt was powerlessness. No matter what was said or done, it was out of the family's hands. No amount of pleading or negotiating worked. No method of trying to control the situation made her parent stop using the substance that would eventually take their life. She felt vulnerable and out of control.

Powerlessness and helplessness can cause us to be more susceptible to anxiety, stress, and depression. Acknowledging that we can't control the actions of anyone else can open space for surrendering the outcome and attaining peace about what is *outside* of our control without sacrificing the care of what is *inside* of our control. I know this isn't easy and takes practice. In further conversation about the experience with her parent, Kim said, "Giving up the control gives you back the power."

I love this reminder from Jeff Brown, author of *Hearticulations*: "It's not like changing a tire. You can influence and support others in their transformation, but you can't change anyone. If there is any learning that I wish had been sealed in my brain at a young age, it is this one. How much time we waste trying to change others, when the only one we can change is staring at us in the mirror."

## Acknowledgment: The Burden

I stalled writing this section for weeks. I knew it was an important one, but it brings back feelings that I used to carry with regard to my mom's mental illness. I had moved through these feelings many years ago, and it wasn't easy. So I didn't relish the thought of allowing them to resurface. They're related to the feeling of being burdened.

A "burden" is anything we have to bear or put up with. It's a heavy load that might involve work, duty, responsibility, or sorrow. When my mother was mentally unwell, I felt the burden of having a mother whose symptoms had created an unstable, unpredictable, and tumultuous dynamic.

One story comes to mind from when I was a young teenager. The home phone landline rang, and my mom answered. No one was on the other end. The phone rang a moment later. But that time, I answered. It was my best friend, Linda. My mom was always pleasant with Linda if she called to speak directly to my mother. But when Linda asked for me, my mom was sometimes moody about it. Linda hung up the phone that day because she was scared to speak to my mother.

Mom asked if Linda had just hung up on her. Out of fear, Linda's response was "No!" I conveyed this to my mother, but she screeched "LIAAAAARRRRR!!!!" in an angry voice loud enough that Linda could hear.

Because of incidents like this, I felt the burden of not having a "normal" mother. Feeling embarrassed and always walking on eggshells, I was angry for the way my friends were treated compared to how I was treated when my mom was in a "mood." I resented her illness. In my view at the time, it wasn't fair that I couldn't just be a regular kid. What if people found out my mom was mentally ill?

Years later, understanding and time healed my old wounds. In fact, Linda, who is still one of my best friends, can find the humor in that incident from when we were younger. Linda and I still call out "LIAAAAARRRRR" every now and again as a joke.

It's natural to feel burdened when a loved one experiences mental health decline. Denying this only adds to our stress, while acknowledging it helps to take the edge off the situation. There's no reason to feel guilty for having such feelings.

### Awareness and Acknowledgment: Compassion Fatigue

Compassion fatigue, also referred to as vicarious trauma, means the negative emotions we can feel when we help others. We may experience changes in our mood, for example, and we might become detached from others or the activities we used to enjoy. We can experience nightmares, excessive worrying, and sleep issues. We can become hypervigilant or on "high alert," staying stuck in a state of fight or flight. The feeling of walking on eggshells around our loved one is also a symptom of compassion fatigue.

There's no question that it's traumatizing to witness your loved one going through a mental well-being breakdown. There might be physical altercations, abusive language, shouting, damage of property, and/or risks to safety.

Recently, I watched a TV show called *Intervention*. They take the viewer on a journey along with real life people who are going through a substance use crisis. At the end of the show, they gather a room full of friends and family members to hold the intervention. Before the loved one who is going through the crisis arrives, the therapist leading the intervention prepares the group as to what to expect. At the end, the person is encouraged to go into rehab and continue their road to recovery. The therapist also tells the group that they, too, are on their own road to recovery from the experience.

It's a great reminder that we're all impacted by these situations, even viewers! In fact, prior to watching shows of this nature, I check in with myself, and sometimes, I feel too vulnerable to witness the pain of others. If I'm not feeling well myself or don't have the emotional capacity, I flip to another channel. Even reading this book can stir up emotions for you, so please be gentle with yourself. Please acknowledge that you may be experiencing compassion fatigue, so practice the self-care you'll read about in the chapters that follow.

## ACKNOWLEDGMENT AND ACTION: GOOD GRIEF

When a loved one dies because of a mental illness, we give ourselves permission to grieve. But we can also grieve for the hopes and dreams we had for our loved one. We might experience anticipatory grief when we fear they might die by suicide if something doesn't change. So grieve the person you knew, remembering the truth of who they are because their symptoms can cloud that.

The five stages of grief were developed by Dr. Elisabeth Kübler-Ross and became famous after she published her book, *On Death and Dying*, in 1969. The five stages are denial, anger, bargaining, depression, and acceptance. Although there are many more stages, these are the main ones. They aren't linear, as they can be felt any time and in any order. They can also carry on to some degree for years.

Grief is both about acknowledging our feelings and allowing ourselves to mourn (grief in action). It's a deeply personal and unique experience for everyone. The grieving process is an important part of healing and learning to adjust to a changing life. All changes bring loss. First and foremost, it's important to acknowledge your feelings and give yourself time and space to grieve.

Grief therapy is an excellent option. As Melody Beattie writes in her book, *The Grief Club: The Secret to Getting Through All Kinds of Change*, being part of the "grief club" of losing a loved one to mental illness is a sacred experience.

## ACCEPTANCE: SURRENDERING

Some people think that surrender is the same as giving up, but it's actually letting go of an outcome that may not be possible. Surrender is the act of yielding to the circumstances and accepting the reality of what is.

In *The Book of Awakening*, author Mark Nepo teaches us that *surrender* is like when a fish goes with the current of the river, and *acceptance* is when the fish is in that flow, runs into a stone, and accepts the situation.

He says we must accept where we are before we can start to figure out how to get out of that place and improve our situation.

Here's an example: I had a bump on my nose for a few years. I thought it was due to my glasses rubbing against it. I just put up with it, thinking there was nothing I could do about it. I was in denial even though my intuition kept telling me to get it checked out. Finally, I made an appointment with a dermatologist and was diagnosed with a form of skin cancer called basal cell carcinoma, which needed to be surgically removed. Understandably, since I have a family history of cancer and my mom had died of cancer, I was full of fear. I could no longer pretend it wasn't there or will it away. If left alone, it could affect my nerves and bones.

I'm not a fan of surgery, so my anxiety levels went through the roof, especially since the spot was on my face and so close to my eyes. But I had to accept reality because I didn't have control over the situation.

Surrender and acceptance can open the doors to the hope and faith we need. It can bring us comfort, as we stop fighting against what is.

## Acceptance: The Blame Game

When someone is going through a mental well-being decline, they tend to blame themselves or others, while the people in their life may blame them for their condition. Sometimes, people even believe they're being punished for something.

After a particular bipolar episode, where the symptomatic behaviors were especially heart-wrenching, my mom shared with me that she couldn't control the behaviors or feelings. She didn't want to do or say those things. Although I had compassion for what she was going through and knew the reason why she was behaving that way, it still wasn't okay for me to be treated like that. So even though your loved one can't control their behaviors, remember that *you* are also not responsible for how they feel or act.

Along with the signs and symptoms that people experience, they tend to have an internal dialogue of "I'm not good enough, there's something wrong with me, and people must think I'm weird or have a character defect." But a mental illness doesn't define us. It isn't who we are. We wouldn't say "you *are* cancer" to someone. We know the cancer isn't who they are. So playing the blame game is counterproductive to everyone involved. We have to come to a place of acceptance (the third of the As) about the reality of the situation without pointing fingers.

## Acknowledgment and Acceptance: Disappointment

Disappointment is the negative emotion we feel when an outcome doesn't match up to our expectations. This might make us feel sad, angry, and frustrated. Disappointment is an unavoidable part of life, but it isn't easy to deal with.

Years ago, a group of friends and I often planned outings, movies, dinners, sleepovers, and travel together. This required coordinating everyone's schedule, as well as advance ticket purchases, deposits, or payments in full for bookings. One of the friends canceled several times at the last minute. This pattern caused lost money, frustration, hurt feelings, and disappointment for the group. Sometime later, this person disclosed that the reason for their cancellations was social anxiety. It was a relief to hear it was nothing personal, and we felt empathy for them. But knowing the cause of the behavior didn't take away the feelings of disappointment. At the end of the day, we still didn't get to spend the fun time together that had been planned with our friend.

It's natural to feel disappointed when a mental health problem prevents someone from partaking of activities. Give yourself permission (without feeling guilty) to have those natural emotions, and remember it isn't a reflection of how you feel about your loved one. It's the illness, *not* the person.

## Awareness, Acknowledgment, and Action: The Pity Party

Welcome to the pity party, where we dance with victim mentality. This is a mindset in which we see ourselves as a victim of negative circumstances. In some cases, victim mentality happens because we've been the victim of wrongdoing by others or have otherwise suffered misfortune through no fault of our own. But the term is also used to describe the tendency to blame our misfortunes on somebody else or on fate.

Victim mentality may manifest itself in a range of different behaviors or ways of thinking, such as:

- Identifying others as the cause for an undesired situation and denying personal responsibility for our own life or circumstances
- Attributing negative intentions to the offender
- Believing that other people are generally more fortunate
- Gaining relief from feeling pity for ourselves or receiving sympathy from others
- Consistent feelings of pessimism, self-pity, and repressed anger[1]

When you're feeling down or stuck, it's tempting to dive into victim mentality. And frankly, I'm a firm believer that it's common to experience waves of it when you're dealing with a loved one facing mental illness. The key, however, is to avoid pulling up a chair and sitting in victim mentality for too long. In fact, visualize musical chairs!

Recognize that victim mentality comes at a hefty price, both mentally and physically. It can leave you feeling drained, and it can build bitterness and resentment. It can also be used as justification for other harmful behaviors, including substance use problems.

We might say, "After what I just went through, I deserve this drink" or "Can't beat 'em, so I may as well join 'em." At the end of the day, victim mentality undermines our resilience, making us less equipped to deal well with tough situations as they arise.

I encourage you to become aware of when you find yourself feeling like a victim and acknowledge it. When you do, I invite you to a Pity Party! Visualize three chairs or as many as you'd like, each chair representing the victim mentality party "favors." Perhaps one chair represents irritation, one represents "I've been given lemons, leaving me feeling sour," and one represents "why me?" Dance around them. When the music stops, "sit" in a chair, get comfortable, whine, complain, emote,

---

1. Manasa, "Victim of Circumstances Mentality Holding You? Let's Change," Wealthfulmind.com, January 11, 2022, accessed November 20, 2024, https://wealthfulmind.com/victim-of-circumstances-mentality.

vent, and let it out. Don't edit yourself with your choice of words. This is for you only. When you've vented enough, remove one of the chairs. Start the music again. Then stop it, and sit in the next chair. Scream, shout, and write your feelings in a journal. Get in touch with the emotions it evokes in you. There's no shame in real feelings! Do this until no chairs remain. This is how you take action to relieve victim mentality.

But then leave the party. It isn't meant to be an "all-nighter" and certainly not an everyday occurrence.

## Juicy Bits

The key "A" here is acknowledging that you are part of this picture, and you are affected. When you suppress your emotions, they can reemerge elsewhere in the form of disease (dis-ease) consistent with the mind-body connection.

Your feelings are valid, even when you may have several feelings at the same time. It's okay to feel excited about something good that's happening in your life, and it's okay to feel anxious or angry about what your loved one is going through. Even though you feel they have it "worse," remember that it isn't a competition. My dad often said to my mom, "my back hurts," and she would respond, "my back hurts, too, *and* I have a headache!" I chuckle every time I share this story! We don't need to one-up each other about who has it the worst.

I understand that it might feel counterintuitive to feel your emotions when your loved one is experiencing lots of feelings. But all of us have factors that affect our mental health. Your emotions are also valid, and it's important to name and honor them. The only person who knows what you're going through is you.

## Exercise: Acknowledge Your Feelings

1. Write down the emotional side effects that you may be experiencing as you navigate loving someone with a decline in their mental wellness.

    Example:

    I feel *helpless* when the *depression is preventing them from getting out of bed.*

I feel *angry* when they *drive under the influence of a substance.*

I feel *scared* when they *attempt suicide.*

I feel *anxious* when they *have a panic attack.*

I feel _____ when _____

I feel _____ when _____

2. Write a letter of comfort to yourself. If you find this challenging, imagine that you're writing to a friend or loved one. Show yourself some compassion, empathy, and understanding for what you're going through. Share words of encouragement, hope, and optimism.

CHAPTER FOUR

# "How Do I Make It All Better?"

PEOPLE ALL OVER THE WORLD REPEATEDLY ASK ME, "HOW CAN I MAKE it all better for my loved one who is suffering with mental illness?" I received a comment on social media recently that encapsulates what many of us feel: "I think the hardest part of supporting my loved one is what my role is in it. How do I know when I am supporting and when I am enabling? How do I balance offering encouragement, ideas, and support with allowing them to hit their low or find their motivation? How do I manage my own heartache when I feel so helpless watching them struggle? How do I manage when they simply don't want or can't accept help and support from me?"

Anyone who has been in a situation of caring for a loved one with mental health decline understands all of those concerns. The reality, however, is *support does not mean fixing*. I learned this the hard way.

During the years my mother had cancer, my dad was her main caregiver, and he ran the household. I visited them monthly, spending a few days each time. In the beginning, I would breeze in with my "helpful" ways and organize the kitchen, clean out the refrigerator, shop for groceries, and cook meals. I was proud of myself until one day, my father asked me to stop. He explained that he had a routine that helped him stay focused. When I came in like the wind blowing knickknacks off the windowsill, it took him days to get "back on track."

I never asked how I could be of assistance. I just saw what I felt needed to be done and did it. But in the process, I inadvertently caused more stress in an already challenging situation.

When I visit my dad now, I'm sensitive to his need for independence and routine. I ask if he would like assistance with something, and he doesn't hesitate to ask me for help when he needs it. When I'm in this situation with others, I now ask how I could offer support. If the other person isn't sure what they need, I might offer suggestions, but I don't make assumptions. The experience with my dad taught me that knowing when to help and when not to help is, in fact, helping.

Years later while my mother was in remission, she said, "You saved my life." She was referring to the time right after her diagnosis when I packed up and moved in with my parents. I acknowledged to her that I was a major support for them, but I also knew I hadn't "saved" her. When she did succumb to her cancer sometime later, the little girl inside me wondered why I couldn't indeed save her.

That experience taught me that we can't save anyone, nor is it our job to do so.

Still, the desire to "fix" or "save" will never go away entirely. What's important is that we recognize it and make a different choice that's better for both ourselves and our loved one. I'm resisting the urge right now to go into fix-it mode for you—the reader. I have a genuine desire to "make it all better" for you. I also dealt with that desire in real life while writing this chapter. I received some disturbing news about my brother, who was attacked in his neighborhood, leaving him with a broken nose and arm, black eyes, and exacerbated mental health problems from the trauma. Even with my training and lived experience, the "fixer" inside me wanted to come out, so I had to stop myself and choose actions that weren't about fixing.

When you get that urge to try to "make it all better," think of mental health as the ocean. It's always there. Some days, it's calm with small waves. Other times, there are big waves. No matter what you do, you'll never be able to stop the waves. Instead, you can focus on navigating yourself through it when the water gets rougher.

When I get caught up in wanting to make it all better, I think of *The Serenity Prayer*: "God grant me the serenity to accept the things I cannot change, the courage to change the things I can, and the wisdom to know the difference." We can't control what someone else is experiencing or feeling any more than we can control the waves. What we do have control over is how we choose to respond.

As you struggle with this strong desire to take away someone else's pain, consider *The OTHER Serenity Prayer* by Eleanor Brown: "Please grant me the serenity to stop beating myself up for not doing things perfectly, the courage to forgive myself because I always try my best, and the wisdom to know that I am a good person with a kind heart."

## THE MAMA BEAR

By definition, a mama bear is the mother of bear cubs. The expression is used metaphorically to refer to a person who is very protective of her "children" and will become violent and dangerous if anyone threatens them. I know this mama bear mode well, and sometimes, it surprises me to discover the lengths I will go to be protective.

I'm reminded of a time when my partner's father, Tommy, was living with dementia, and it was dangerous for him to drive. He was furious about losing his independence, and one day, he reached for the car keys. I went into mama bear mode and was prepared to take a punch from him, if necessary. As I swooped in to grab the keys first, he raised his fists. Thankfully, he didn't punch me, and I managed to prevent him from driving.

As you can see, in some circumstances, mama bear mode can be a good thing. We can save a life. But in other situations where life and death aren't involved, mama bear mode can make matters worse.

When I heard about my brother's attack, the mama bear inside me wanted everybody to get out of the way while I put those attackers straight. But would adding to the aggression help the situation? No. Would it take away my brother's physical and mental pain? No. I couldn't change what happened.

Instead, I could look for ways to possibly prevent something like that from happening again. I could show love and support by visiting my brother and offering him comfort and attention. I could also get support for my own feelings about the attack.

## The Problem-Solver

Many moons ago at a boardroom table, a previous boss of mine discussed a challenge the company was experiencing. Without being asked, I gave my opinion and volunteered my services to "fix it." There was a hush in the room. After the meeting, a close colleague took me aside and said, "I understand you want to help, but getting involved when you don't know the full picture and when it's not your place could make the situation worse. Wait to be asked." I had opened a can of worms without realizing it.

In my efforts to be the rescuer, I was perceived as "sticking my oar in where it didn't belong." I was later told that my boss was furious with me. Lesson learned!

If you're the wonderful, caring, hard-to-see-others-in-pain, jump-into-action-and-try-to-solve-the-problem person, try resisting those impulses. We can make a different choice and trust the other person to deal with their problem in their own way. We don't have to take their problem from them. Instead, do your best to understand the person even when their choices may not make sense. Give them enough room to discover for themselves why they feel upset and enough time to determine for themselves what's best. Hold back the desire to give them "good" advice.

## Don't Feed the Animals

Whenever we see a loved one in pain, it's natural to rush to be the savior. We don't trust their ability to help themselves. But what if they're going through the very thing they need in order to grow?

Nature analogies are helpful and easy to remember when I find myself trying to be a savior. For example, they say "don't feed the animals" for a reason. Feeding wildlife does more harm than good. Often, what we feed them isn't nutritionally sound for them, and doing so can create dependence on humans, which only puts them in danger.

My great niece, Ava, shared with me what she learned from Girl Guides outdoor camp. She said that animals have an instinctive way of managing a forest fire. They know how to find food on their own, even in severe conditions like that. It's also true that fire is a natural part of most ecosystems. Even if animals aren't specifically adapted to wildfires, many tend to do better in the aftermath. As trees burn away, they create open access for sunlight to hit the ground, helping different types of vegetation grow and providing animals with more food sources.

Sometimes, we think we're "saving" someone, but we actually harm them inadvertently. For instance, if we move a baby bird, its mother might not be able to find it. A caterpillar during transformation looks like it's in distress, pain, and struggle. But it needs to go through the transformation by itself. The struggle to open its cocoon is what builds the strength in its wings. Without the struggle, the emerging new butterfly would lack the strength to fly and would die quickly. The timing of its emergence from the chrysalis is key. So if a well-meaning human interferes and tries to "help" the butterfly with its struggle, that human will no doubt harm the insect.

In other words, we all need to be discerning about the type of help we offer someone else.

## An Inside Job

A longtime friend has been in alcohol recovery for twenty years. I asked him for insight about how to support our mutual friend who is six months into his alcohol-free life. "You do your best to be there for them, listen, offer support, and guide them to other supports," he said. "But at the end of the day, it's really an inside job."

It's hard to see someone in pain, especially someone who is close to us. But it's like the old adage, "You can lead a horse to water, but you can't make it drink." We can provide an opportunity for someone to get help, but we can't force them to take advantage of it.

Think of when a lifeguard approaches a person who is drowning. They employ a firm measure of self-protection by offering a buoy or rope because a drowning person is in a state of panic. It's well documented that this panic can cause them to latch on to the person who is trying to help them and cause that person to drown as well. The lifeguard rule gives permission to let someone drown if it's clear that helping them will drown both people.

If helping someone is dragging you down, you may need to let go and move on to preserve yourself. This helps you eliminate unhealthy forms of helping.

> ## You Are Not *Their* Therapist
>
> When your loved one relies on you for too much emotional support, it's tempting and easy to fall into the trap of taking on the role of their therapist. When you're tempted to do that, stop yourself! This is a conflict of interest, and you aren't a trained mental health professional. Even if you were, it would create an unhealthy dynamic that wouldn't work as a long-term solution. Knowing your boundaries is crucial.
>
> Remember that your role is to listen, give love, and support with empathy. Only a professional mental health counselor or therapist can offer your loved one ways to manage their symptoms.

### IT'S BROKE, BUT DON'T FIX IT

Showing support means not having all the answers. Let's start at the point where you recognized a mental health "problem" with a loved one, colleague, or friend. Perhaps you saw the signs and symptoms of a decline in their mental well-being, or the person told you directly they were going through a problem. In that moment, it might have been tempting to think, "What has worked for me will work for them." Then it's natural to want to offer advice to try to make it all better. You may even want to give them a toolbox full of "fix-it ideas." But there are good reasons not to do that. Television journalist Dan Harris suggests that rather than focusing on the problem and the belief that it needs to be solved, we can focus on the dynamics that the problem creates, which will be easier to manage.

Remember that mental health problems don't define a person. Their behaviors are not who they are. Judging them won't change their behaviors. So rather than judge, which keeps us hyper-focused on the problem, we can strive to accept them and look for ways to love them.

We can accept the reality of the situation. Understand that accepting isn't giving up, settling, or denying what's happening. It just means you understand that it's the reality. As I've mentioned, the Buddhists call this accepting "what is." Accepting is recognizing that life has changed, and you can no longer go back to how it was. It isn't passive; it's defiant. It's a way to rebel against shutting down, living in a destructive environment, or losing hope. In a world that encourages quick fixes and black-and-white thinking, acceptance teaches us the expansive and revolutionary power of embracing the less bright days and all that comes with them.

While you're at it, give *yourself* what psychologists call "radical self-acceptance." Accept everything about yourself, your current situation, and your life without question, blame, or pushback. You can't fail at this. There is no roadmap, no precedent for this, and we're all truly doing the best we can in a challenging situation.

## IT'S OKAY—UMMM... NO, IT'S NOT

"Stop saying it's okay. It's not okay," my mom said in frustration on her deathbed as her body was giving way to breast cancer.

I was the daughter who came into a room like a "breath of fresh air and bright ray of sunshine." In that moment, I didn't know what else to say, but "it's okay!" The urge to make it all better was actually a disservice to my mother and to myself.

It wasn't okay. It sucked. It tore my insides apart.

Mom was in and out of consciousness during this time. In one of her few lucid moments, she asked, "Am I dying?"

Silence. How could I possibly respond to that?

She asked again in a state of panic. "Am I dying?"

"Yes, Mom, you're dying," I answered as gently as I could muster.

"I don't want to die," she said in anguish.

And in my typical "trying to make it feel better fashion," I followed up with, "but you aren't dying right now."

There was nothing wrong with saying that, but just because we say it's okay doesn't mean it is. Let's ditch the pretending and get real. Life can suck at times, so I suggest we at least consider naming it instead of dismissing it to try to make it more digestible.

Emotions need motion. Let's stop pushing them down. If they're in motion, we can release them. For example, if you stuff a beach ball under water, what happens? It can only go so far, and when you let go, it comes right back up to the surface with force. When we feel emotions, pushing them down and trying to control them can result in an overwhelming outburst that does more harm than good.

Again, let's not judge the reason for tears. Let's just allow them to flow. They're healthy. Keep reminding yourself that crying releases "feel good chemicals" that help to manage both physical and emotional pain.

When my mother was told that her breast cancer had spread to her liver, and there were no further treatments for her, she looked at me, my dad, and my partner and said, "Okay, let's all have a good cry."

In my experience, the tears do eventually stop. There are no guidelines for how much crying is too much, however. A study in the 1980s found that women cry an average of 5.3 times per month, and men cry an average of 1.3 times per month. A newer study found that the average duration for a crying session is eight minutes. (If you're concerned that you're crying too much, if you can't seem to stop crying, or have started crying more than usual, talk to your doctor. It may be a sign of depression or another mood disorder.)

## Vulnerability Hangover

When someone tells you about their mental well-being decline, they might ignore you the next time you see them. Maybe you've spent hours listening to a loved one's feelings, hearing about their challenging times and dark days. Perhaps you've encouraged them to seek professional support. Then the next day, you check in on them, but they don't return your calls or texts. You bump into them at the store, but they barely make eye contact. This is what is often referred to as a "vulnerability hangover."

When that happens, we tend to blame ourselves: *Did I say something wrong? Did I overstep?* But this has nothing to do with what you said or did. It's a common occurrence when someone feels extra sensitive and vulnerable.

Opening up can feel extremely exposing, leaving the person feeling drained, embarrassed, and even regretful that they told you so much. They may be thinking, "They must think I'm weird or that something's wrong with me."

I suggest meeting them where they are. Continue to build rapport and trust, and go at their pace, not yours. Get rid of your agenda, and release the desire to act on your possible preconceived notions of what's best for them. They may need time to process and heal before they speak with you again.

What you don't want to do is make them your project. Don't hunt them down and ask if they contacted the professional you found. Don't lecture them, and don't "should" them—telling them what they "should" do.

In his memoir, *Friends, Lovers, and the Big Terrible Thing*, Matthew Perry, the late actor from the *Friends* TV show, acknowledged the amount of self-loathing that tagged along during his mental health crisis. "Shoulding" and lecturing can sometimes elicit more self-loathing in people who are experiencing mental health problems.

## The Doubt

*Did I say the right thing? Am I going to upset them? Who am I to try to help anybody?* Have you had any of those thoughts? When supporting someone through a mental well-being decline, you might feel like you're walking on eggshells, not knowing how the person will respond or if you've said the right thing.

One of my best friends, Linda, had a challenging experience like this. Her neighbor found their partner dead from suicide and ran over to Linda's for help. She felt overwhelmed and unsure of what to say in such a dire situation. But she said she heard my voice in her head from my course, saying "If you don't remember the A.L.G.E.S. (Assess/Assist, Listen Non-Judgmentally/Give Reassurance/Encourage Supports/Self-Care for the First Aider) in the moment, remember the 'L' for Listening Non-Judgmentally, and connect as a fellow human heart to heart." She listened, she didn't give advice, she didn't act all-knowing, she didn't try to fix the problem, she didn't take it on as her own problem, and she didn't try to take away their pain. She simply listened.

When we *really* listen, the other person feels heard. They know they matter, and that can make a world of difference. How often do any of us get someone else's full attention? Let's do more of that!

## Juicy Bits
### Memorize These Three Cs and Gs
**Cs:** I didn't **cause** it. I can't **control** it. I can't **cure** it.
**Gs: Get** off their back. **Get** out of the way. **Get** on with your own life.

I got a call from a loved one looking for support with a significant other who was going through a mental well-being decline. After listening non-judgmentally, we came to a standstill about what to do next. I said, "Be in care of yourSELF. What do YOU need right now? How can you support yourself right now?"

Start with the SELF. What are YOU feeling? How are you managing your feelings? How is this situation impacting you? What support do YOU need?

## Exercises to Avoid "Fix It" Mode
Trying to "make it all better" for your loved one isn't an easy habit to change. It takes practice. Let's get in tune with when you have a tendency to jump into fix-it mode, and let's choose another response.

1. Think of a time you jumped right into action to "fix" how your loved one was feeling or what they were enduring. Write down how you felt about that experience. What were some of the emotions that came up for you then and now as you remember it.

2. What did you learn from the experience about your desire to fix it?

3. What might you do differently if it were to happen again?

4. Finally, I invite you to write in your journal about your desire to fix your loved one's mental health problems. What would you love to say to the problem, disorder, or behaviors? Write down what you truly feel about it all. After you've emptied it out in your journal, place your hands on your heart to appreciate the fact that you care so deeply. Give yourself thanks for wanting to make a difference in the life of your loved one, and remind yourself that your job is to be supportive, not a fixer or savior.

Chapter Five

# Help Me Help You Help Me

In May 2019, one of my worst nightmares came true. I was staying at our family home before a speaking event in Ottawa. Around midnight, I was awakened by a couple of loud banging sounds. As I leaped out of bed, I knew intuitively that my father had fallen. I ran to the top of the stairs and yelled down, "Dad, did you fall?"

Bracing myself for the answer, I heard a soft "yes." I raced down the stairs to find him at the bottom of the landing where the stairs met the basement door. He had been carrying a large pile of towels and tripped over a grandchild's toy that hadn't been put away.

He was in the fetal position with his head resting on the towels that gathered like a pillow. If I didn't know any better, I would have thought he was purposely taking a rest. "I'm going to let things settle before I get up," he said.

Luckily, there were no broken bones (phew!), but his shin took a beating. The days that followed, however, his leg swelled up, and he could barely walk on it. Mom and I kept insisting he go to the doctor and get it checked out. But we were met with "I'll be fine; I'm not going to the doctors. What are they going to do? It just needs time to heal." No amount of pleading, coercing, or negotiating worked.

I was full of anxiety and feeling desperate. Despite our home remedies, Dad's leg was getting worse and worse. I knew he needed professional help, but expressing anger, frustration, or becoming demanding would only have made him more resistant. Finally, I asked him, "Dad, if this was me, what would you tell me to do?" In that instant, he picked up the phone.

When we want to help another person, it can be difficult to know the best approach. "What if I say the wrong thing?" "What if they resist support and/or they say they're going to get support but don't?"

To truly support someone, "help me help you" is a powerful approach. Do you remember the scene from the movie *Jerry Maguire*, where Tom Cruise says to Cuba Gooding Jr., "Help me help you"? When we come from a place of curiosity rather than jumping to a solution, we put ourselves in a better position to make a real difference for someone else.

The final "help me" in the title of this chapter means that the person who needs help from you is, in turn, helping you learn what to do for them. And in helping you help them, they are also helping you be of service, which is nurturing to your own mental health. (Of course, I say this with the caveat that you don't want to *over*-help someone, as we've already discussed.)

When you approach your loved one with genuine concern and care, they will feel that. Be mindful, however, that some people don't feel comfortable speaking about mental health issues. Take into consideration their social beliefs, culture, and environment.

Effective support can also involve sitting beside someone without speaking a word. You can simply be present and provide a safe space for them just to be. When I don't feel good, it's counterproductive when someone else tries to "make" me feel better. By connecting as an authentic fellow human being heart to heart and by truly listening, we provide excellent support.

With these points in mind, let's dive into more things to consider while supporting another through a mental well-being decline and some of the ways you can communicate your concern and encourage other support.

## You Are Not Alone

First of all, I understand that you may feel like you're alone, but you aren't. According to the National Institutes of Health, there is evidence in the world today of the negative impact of mental disorders on the health and well-being of family caregivers. It's often reported to be worse in cases of depressive disorders or embarrassing behaviors.[1]

When someone is going through a mental well-being decline, it can feel like no one else knows what they're going through or what you're going through. What they need is relatability, empathy, compassion, grace, and understanding so that they don't feel alone. Chances are they're already experiencing self-loathing, despising how they feel and how it makes others feel around them. Listening to them non-judgmentally can do wonders and even sometimes ease their symptoms.

At the same time, you must recognize that it isn't up to you to change their behaviors. Remember that they have to do that themselves!

The most effective way to guide someone toward recovery is to match your encouragement, empathy, and support to the stage they're in. Let's look at the Stages of Change so that you can determine where your loved one falls on that spectrum.

## THE STAGES OF CHANGE

The Stages of Change process was developed by Prochaska and DiClemente in the late 1970s. It's a model (also referred to as The Transtheoretical Theory) that allows health care professionals to meet the client where they are in their readiness to change.[2] Although your loved one is not your "client," awareness of where they fall within the Stages of Change will give you insight as to the best approach. The following is a list of the various stages and suggested ways to support your loved one in each:

### *Stage 1.* **Precontemplation:** *Not ready to change*

At this stage, the person may not even be aware that they're having a problem with their mental health. If they suspect there is a problem, they tend to minimize it, thinking it isn't serious, or they believe they can handle it on their own. They may not be ready for change.

---

1. J. T. Ndlovu and K. E. Mokwena, "Burden of Care of Family Caregivers for People Diagnosed with Serious Mental Disorders in a Rural Health District in Kwa-Zulu-Natal, South Africa," *Healthcare* (Basel) 11, no. 19 (October 2023), 2686, doi:10.3390/healthcare11192686.

2. "Transtheoretical Model," Wikipedia, accessed December 8, 2024, https://en.wikipedia.org/wiki/Transtheoretical_model.

Pushing someone who isn't ready to seek help may be counterproductive and frustrating for all involved. It's better to focus on all the benefits they could expect from support and ask them to share which benefits would be most important to them.

***Stage 2*. Contemplation:** *Getting ready to change*
At this stage, the person is starting to recognize that they have a problem and thinking about making changes. You might hear them say, "I have a problem, and I think I need to do things differently." It's common for people to remain in this stage for quite some time, tossing between the pros and cons of getting professional help. You can support them by discussing how the behaviors are getting in the way of the life they want to live. You can help them visualize how their life would be better if they sought help. Discuss with them how their pros outweigh their cons.

***Stage 3*. Preparation:** *Ready to change*
At this stage, they are aware that the advantages of getting support outweigh the positives of continuing on their own. Continue to be supportive and encouraging. Help them create a plan and follow through. Work together to find professional and other supports, and let them know they can reach out to you as they go through the process.

***Stage 4*. Treatment:** *Taking action*
At this stage, the person has committed to getting support. Continue to be patient and understanding. Cheer them on as they adopt new positive behaviors. Help coordinate dates for professional support, and perhaps encourage positive changes by driving them to appointments. Some people prefer company along the way.

***Stage 5*. Recovery:** *Maintaining changes*
In this stage, the person is fully engaged and committed to their new behaviors and treatment. Remind them that even with a diagnosis, they can still live a happy, healthy, and functioning life.

## Demystifying Therapy

Of course, therapy is the number one recommendation for support. You may be tempted to present the person with a treatment plan without fully understanding their situation. But researching treatments without your loved one's input should only be a last resort. It's better to explore options together, and it's important to acknowledge that choosing to go to therapy can feel scary and overwhelming.

Some people may even believe that a therapist will tell them what to do to "solve" their problem. You can encourage your loved one by emphasizing that therapy gives them someone who will provide undivided attention with empathy and no interruptions, as well as professional guidance about what they're experiencing. Let them know that healthy people seek therapy every day to improve the quality of their lives.

Going to therapy was a life-changer for me, and to this day, I still enjoy its benefits.

## The "Advice-or"

As you offer your own support to your loved one, it's helpful to remember that "good" advice is relative. What may be good for you may not be for them. Resist the urge to tell them what they "should" do. I often say, "Don't let anyone 'should' on you today, and don't 'should' on yourself."

Remember that when you jump into "fix it" mode, the other person can feel unheard and even rejected. You may be trying to sort out the details (the who, what, when, and where), and you may not be aware of the feelings or emotions behind their words. After all, most of us were never taught how to describe or name our feelings. So they might not be able to communicate what's going on with them. Rather than jump in with solutions, remind yourself to ask questions and listen.

Brené Brown's informative, human-centered TV series *Atlas of the Heart* dives deep into defining emotions, feelings, and the words we use to describe them. I suggest watching this to become more insightful about your own feelings, as well as the emotions of others, especially if you're supporting a loved one in mental well-being decline.

Then I suggest that you listen carefully to your loved one before ever offering any advice. As a psychotherapist, you may assume that I'm naturally a great listener, but I'm not! I have needed a lot of practice. I have to work against thinking of a response before the other person has finished speaking, which only creates disconnection. If there is a pause, my natural inclination would be to jump in with the word I think they want to say, but 90 percent of the time, I'm wrong! As a result, the person may feel rushed, thinking, "I'd better hurry, or I won't be able to get a word in edgewise," or they might shut down and disengage. Truly listening provides an environment where the person can show up authentically with more of an opportunity to be heard without assumptions and receive our support.

> *"Most people experiencing distressing emotions and thoughts want an empathetic listener before being offered helpful options and resources."*
> —MENTAL HEALTH FIRST AID USA MANUAL

## USE YOUR BORN TOOLS

Do you read operating manuals, or do you just start using the gadget or tool? I have a tendency to skip the instructions! For example, my cellphone has all kinds of capabilities that I've never known about. The truth is that we all have natural born tools available to us, and perhaps we underestimate them. So let's dive into our human tools for listening and communicating non-judgmentally.

**Listen with your ears.** You may have heard the adage that we were born with two ears and one mouth. All the more to listen with. You can't speak and listen at the same time.

**Listen with your eyes.** Make gentle eye contact. Don't stare. In some cultures, direct eye contact can be a sign of disrespect. Stay focused on the other person, and avoid distractions like your cellphone.

**Listen with your mind.** Let go of preconceived ideas about what you think your loved one is thinking. Keep your mind open, even if you suspect you will dislike what you are about to hear. Learn to concentrate on the moment, and clear your mind of distractions. I often find myself drifting off to a response or memory trigger, so I have to keep bringing myself back to the present moment and resist that urge to wander. It isn't easy and takes practice!

**Listen with your heart.** Be concerned for and genuinely interested in the person to whom you are listening. That will speak louder than anything you actually say.

*"It may be good to speak in such a way that others love to listen to you, but it's better to listen in such a way that others love to speak to you."*
—Anonymous

## Rescuing: Help That Doesn't Help

We've talked about rescuing and "fix it" mode, but I understand it might still be difficult to discern the difference between helping and rescuing. Let's discuss that a bit more. When you rescue, you rob the other person of the opportunity to grow. By attempting to rescue, we disempower the other person. For example, let's say that it seems like everywhere you turn, there are problems. Your friend is struggling with a breakup, your partner is fighting with his boss, and your daughter has a mental illness. You're worried and concerned, and you feel the need to step in to help. Here's what it might look like when you are in *rescue* mode:

*Your belief is that they will get better with your support and by following your advice. You call or text your friend several times a day to see how they're feeling, and you research and send an article about how to manage a breakup. You tell your partner to meet with his boss, and you tell him what to say and how to act. You check in with your daughter hourly, and you look up the medication she's on, as well as its side effects. You attempt to call her doctor to discuss a better medication in case she doesn't feel better soon.*

Here's what it might look like when you are in *helping* mode:

*You ask how you can best support each person, and you listen to what they need. You allow them to do their own research and make their own phone calls, and you only provide the support they ask for.*

## Use Your Voice

On a recent trip with my elderly father to Ireland, a computer mix-up with our airplane seats meant I would no longer be sitting next to him, and he wouldn't have the extra leg room he needed. We had paid for these special seats months in advance! My father was adamant that he needed me to assist him with his medical needs on the flight, and he was absolutely right.

As you can imagine, I was in a state of panic. Recognizing that I was in need of support, my dad's local assistant (who had helped him onto the plane) asked me in her Irish accent, "What's the matter, pet?" After explaining the situation, she suggested I take a deep breath and ask the flight attendants to help arrange the seats to accommodate our requirements. She said, "Use your voice. That's what it's there for!" I appreciated the reminder. It made the world of difference, and we did get it all sorted.

When you're in a position to be an advocate in a healthy way for your loved one, speak up! Use your voice, and ask for the support the two of you need. You may be surprised how many people will be willing to help.

### The Problem-Solving Brain

It's difficult to avoid "fixing," even when we ask our loved one, "Do you want my advice, or would you prefer I just listen to you?" We're full of good intentions and find it difficult to prevent our problem-solving brains from looking for answers. Chances are, your loved one can feel that!

So instead, consider asking, "Do you want me to give you advice, or do you want me to understand you?" This signals your problem-solving brain to go into "understanding" mode instead.

When we give advice before we understand someone fully, we make assumptions based on our own experience more than the other person's experience. By listening to understand, we basically say, "I believe in you and want to hear where you're coming from." That feels better to both the listener and the speaker. Can you feel the difference?

### It's Not About the Nail

A client of mine shared a video with me that poked fun at our "fix it" desires. This ninety-second video, *It's Not About the Nail*, by Jason Headley,[3] is a blatant scenario of what most of us tend to do in a listening/supportive role. The woman in the video has a big nail sticking out of

---

3. Jason Headley, "It's Not About the Nail," YouTube, accessed December 9, 2024, https://www.youtube.com/watch?v=-4EDhdAHrOg.

her head. In this situation, let's consider "the nail" to represent the mental health problem or illness. Her complaints are all related to the nail ("there's pressure in my head; I can't sleep"). Every time her loved one suggests that removing the nail would fix her, she says, "It's not about the nail!" and gets angry at him for not listening to her. She's upset about what's she going through and needs emotional support from her partner. But her partner is desperately trying to solve the problem for her.

This leaves the support-seeking person frustrated because they don't feel heard. The support-providing person is also frustrated because they just don't understand why she won't simply take their advice and fix it.

Even with a "nail" sticking out of our head, we might need to express our feelings and have them validated. It's possible she didn't yet understand that the nail was causing her problem. Sometimes, people fear that the solution to the problem will cause worse pain or be a waste of time. So accept their perspective. They're feeling pain and hoping you can soothe it by really listening.

People want to be heard for very simple reasons:

*They need to express how they feel.*

*They need to feel supported.*

*They need to feel they aren't alone.*

*They need to believe their feelings are valid.*

*They need to feel that their voice matters to someone.*

*They need to speak out loud to help them understand their own feelings.*

Of course, the caveat to this is if your loved one is at risk of harming themselves or others, the situation becomes more urgent and needs to be acted upon immediately. Certainly, a literal nail in the head requires a rush to the emergency room!

## THE FINE LINE

When listening to someone in a supportive way, you may say something like, "When I (or family member, loved one, friend, etc.) went through something similar, I found it helpful to do _____." This provides relatability and gives your loved one the awareness that others have gone through a similar experience. I say "similar" because as cliché as it sounds, no two snowflakes are alike. As I mentioned previously, your experience is not theirs and vice versa.

Still, sharing your own experience can provide hope, optimism, and comfort that they aren't alone. It can help them focus on how to feel better without the extra burden of "stinkin' thinkin'"—the internal dialogue and self-stigma that can directly interfere with our healing journey.

What you don't want to do is be that person who says, "I know exactly how you feel" and then proceed to take over the conversation with stories of what you went through, leaving them feeling dismissed.

## JUDGING THE JUDGER

When I learned about listening and communicating non-judgmentally, I realized I'd been so *judgy*! I share this with you as a cautionary tale because I suddenly started to judge myself for being judgmental! Then I started to recognize the judgments of others. We can stop this cycle *of judging the judger who judges the judge!* See where I'm going here?

I believe we all have a big red imaginary RESET button, and we have the ability to press it at any time. When you find yourself being judgmental, press that RESET button and choose another way. Have grace and compassion for yourself. The key is that you are now aware and can make another choice.

## DON'T BE THE JOURNALIST

It may be tempting to think you need all the facts before you can help someone. I can relate to that tendency. The "fixer" in me wants to know exactly what I'm dealing with so that I can find the perfect solution. But stop the presses! In order to support someone, you don't need the who, what, when, whys, or "then what happened." It's more beneficial to avoid getting caught up in the "drama" of it all. The full "story" isn't necessary to get to the heart of the matter.

When someone goes through a traumatic experience, speaking about the trauma can do more harm than good. It can be re-triggering and possibly create re-injury. Of course, if the person wants to speak about what happened, let them, even if they repeat themselves. But otherwise, focus on the signs, symptoms, and opportunities to support them.

If you've known them a long time, however, you might remind them what worked for them in the past. All of us have been through challenges. To overcome them, chances are we've used support systems, inner strength, perseverance, courage, and persistence. Reminding the person what they've previously come through and what helped them before can be useful. We all tend to forget.

## SUPPORT THROUGH QUESTIONS

Nevertheless, I do encourage you to ask questions to get a better understanding of what someone is thinking or feeling. Sometimes, to avoid jumping to conclusions, we need more detail/context, but only if they want to share it.

Ask simple, open-ended questions. Ask how your loved one has been doing and feeling. You can encourage them to expand on their answer by acknowledging some of the changed behaviors you've noticed. Let them know you care and are concerned about the changes.

To discern what kind of support someone may need, here are some suggested supportive and non-judgmental questions that people going through a mental well-being decline often wish we'd ask.

"What do you mean by _____?"

"When we were talking before, you mentioned that you've been dealing with [insert issue/concern/event]. Can you tell me more about this?"

"When you say that you don't care about anything anymore, do you mean you feel disengaged from your hobbies and work? Do you mean from friends and family as well or something else?"

"I've noticed you aren't as engaged on social media/quit the lacrosse team/lost interest in your walking group/have been sleeping more/have been calling in sick to work more frequently. How are you feeling these days?" Be curious and caring; be mindful not to come from a place of interrogation.

"How would you like things to be different?" I know I'm harping on this, but it's so important: don't assume they want to be "fixed." Find out what they'd like for themselves.

"*What's the underlying pain?*" There may be something else underneath the behavior, such as a negative belief about themselves like, "I'm a failure" or "I'm not good enough."

"*Would it surprise you to know that when someone goes through an experience like this, it's common to feel _____?*" They may not be aware others have had similar experiences, so they might be comforted to know they aren't alone.

"*Are you getting enough sleep? How's your appetite?*" Some basic human needs can be affected by mental illness. They may not even be aware of how these issues have impacted them.

"*I know you recently had some changes at school/had a divorce in the family/lost your job/lost a loved one. Is there anything you'd like to get off your mind?*" Give them the space to share without jumping in.

"*I care about you. How can I help you through this?*" They may have something in mind. If they say they don't know, ask, "If you did know, what would it be?" They will usually come up with something. "I don't know" tends to be a knee-jerk reaction.

"*When is the best time to check in with you again?*" The world is full of good intentions, but if we don't put a time on our calendar, it may never happen. Pencil it in with flexibility in case you need to reschedule.

"*Want to hang out, maybe go for a coffee? Or watch that Netflix series we've been wanting to see? Or we could make our favorite meal together.*" Sometimes, when we are always in our "stuff," we just need a breather from it. A good distraction used in moderation can be helpful as long as it isn't the go-to way of coping.

"*Do you have any errands or tasks I can do for you? Can I pick up the kids from school or put the laundry away?*" Giving suggestions helps take the pressure off your loved one to have to think how you can help. Just be sure you're able to do what you offer without feeling obliged, and remember not to jump in to do these things without verifying it's truly what they need and want.

"*Have you reached out to anyone, such as calling a helpline, doctor, or family?*" See if you can find out what help they have already sought. If they've done that already, and you suggest it, they might feel frustrated. If they have sought support, ask them more information about their experience. Again, of course, be mindful not to interrogate.

*"Would you like me to assist looking up some information and resources for you?"* While you do this, you might find some useful information for yourself as well!

## THE PARAPHRASE AND THE PARROT

*Paraphrasing* or summarizing is a great way to show the person you're there to support them, especially if you follow it with validation of their feelings. Below are some examples:

"What I hear you saying is that work has been challenging. You've been arguing more with your wife, and you're looking to go to couples counseling. To top it all off, your furnace stopped working, and you aren't sure how you'll come up with the funds for the repair. All that can be stressful. It's natural to feel overwhelmed. I imagine I would feel the same way."

"From what you've told me about having overwhelming negative thoughts, would it surprise you to know that when people experience the same, they also have problems with their sleep and concentration? Would you say the negative thoughts and ruminating have become unmanageable?"

*Parroting* is another conversational technique where the listener repeats what the other person has said word for word, but only the highlights. Some people mistake it for repeating back every word *exactly* like a parrot, but the goal is simply to ensure you've heard them correctly and encourage them to clarify their thoughts, whether you parrot or paraphrase. You simply want to help them feel heard and validated.

When you use these techniques, be careful to use encouraging words. Stay away from negative words or attitudes.

## COMMIT TO THE PROCESS

It's natural to feel hesitant to offer support, especially if you're worried about overstepping. I'm reminded of an experience I had recently. I was driving along a country road, and I saw a deer up ahead. So I slowed down. Aside from all the cars whipping by, the deer didn't hesitate to continue across the road. Luckily, he made it to the other side unharmed. But he committed to getting across. Had he hesitated, he might not have navigated all the cars with such good timing. If I had hesitated and failed to slow down, I surely would have hit the deer.

The message for me was to go for it! The chances are higher that you and your loved one will both come out the other side better for it, even if you end up overstepping and having to course correct. There's more of a risk of harm with hesitation than providing support to someone. Just pay attention to the clues to see if you've offered more than the other person wants and are beginning to overwhelm them.

## When It Rains, It Pours

A few years back, we were setting off on an exciting vacation. I got my hair done in preparation and got all dressed up. Our friends were coming to pick us up in a limousine to take us to the airport. As the limo approached, the skies opened up, and it started to pour with the type of rain that leaves puddles within seconds. With excitement, I opened the door to wave at my friends and let them know we'd be right there. But as I opened the door, our Jack Russell Maggie bolted out and ran down the street. I went right into action and ran after her, as my hairdo got soaked, and my mascara ran down my face. Even my white outfit became see-through!

Maggie went her usual escape route, so I was able to bring her back within minutes. Still, I was soaked from head to toe, and there was no time to change. The skies miraculously cleared after that, and down the driveway came my partner, Dave, with the bags. Once we were all in the limo, we managed a few chuckles about how I looked and how surprising life can be sometimes.

My friend asked Dave why he didn't run out after Maggie, too? "Well, there was no reason for us both to get wet!" he answered. Such wisdom! Here's the point: I managed the situation, and if I had needed help, I would have asked. Both of us didn't need to get drenched!

When you include yourself in your loved one's situation, stay mindful of your own mental health. It will allow you to show up stronger, more authentic, and create a safe space for them to express themselves.

Their behaviors might cause you to go through your own challenges without the emotional or mental resources to fully support them. You aren't obliged to be a resource for every single person you know. It's okay to say something like, "I'm not the best person to speak about this with you. I do care and support you. I know there are times when we need someone to listen and when we need to be the listener. Perhaps I can help you find someone else who can listen." This is still providing support.

## THE EMPATHIZER

Often, people get confused about the difference between empathy and sympathy.

Sympathy is feeling *for* someone as best we can relate, but it's pity and can sound condescending in certain contexts. It doesn't help us build deep connections with others. Instead, it only offers surface-level understanding.

Empathy is feeling *with* someone. It builds connection. It's doing our best to understand what they're going through, not what we *think* they're going through. You may be familiar with the saying, "put yourself in their shoes." That's empathy.

I affectionately refer to Brené Brown as the "Empathy Queen." She suggests we take it a step further and walk beside them as they walk in their *own* shoes. We will never know, even if we've had similar experiences, what it's like to walk in their shoes. Only they really know. So empathy isn't connecting to an experience; it's connecting to the emotions underneath the experience.

Having empathy is key. So do your best not to jump in with "at least" statements. For example, if someone tells you they're getting a divorce, don't respond with, "well, *at least* you got married." Some might find such a comment funny, but it will be hurtful to someone who's in pain. A more empathetic response would be, "Thank you for sharing that with me. Please help me understand what you're going through."

In order for us to be empathetic, we have to attempt to see the world as others see it or see it from their perspective as best we can. Use the techniques in this chapter to communicate your understanding of the other person's feelings.

## What Does It Mean?

When a loved one is going through a challenging time, we tend to internalize, become a little sensitive, and potentially make it about us. But it isn't a reflection on you. Don't make it mean something it doesn't. For example, if your loved one is angry and speaking aggressively, you may think you've done something to upset them. You may think it's your fault. So ask them what it's about. They might just be having a rough day.

When asking supportive questions of your loved one, you may not like what they feel or say. You may not know what to do with their answer. Simply do your best not to personalize what's happening or feel inadequate if you aren't sure what to do.

## Listening Fatigue

When you truly listen, it takes energy and can be tiring. It may also stir up emotions for you or trigger memories of previous experiences. So self-care is an integral part of being an effective listener.

When you are thanked for listening, accept the gift of gratitude, and let the other person know you're happy it was helpful. This also reassures them they haven't burdened you with their problems.

When supporting someone who is experiencing a mental health difficulty, use it as an opportunity to practice listening as a receiver rather than as a critic or problem-solver. Practice understanding them rather than achieving agreement from them or trying to change them.

*"To be fully seen by somebody, then, and to be loved anyhow—this is a human offering that can border on miraculous."*

—Elizabeth Gilbert

## Careless Whispers

Have you thought or said some of the below statements to someone who may be going through a mental well-being decline? If so, I invite you to have compassion and grace for both yourself *and* your loved one. As Maya Angelou says, "Do the best you can until you know better. Then when you know better, do better." Reading this book is a great way to learn, overcome, improve, and grow. My hope for you is that you'll recognize that thinking or saying some of these can be counterproductive:

"Just snap out of it."
"Get over yourself."
"You need to get out more and stop wallowing."
"Just think—things could be so much worse."
"You really have nothing to worry about."
"Stop complaining; things aren't that bad all the time."
"It isn't as bad as you think."
"You're always so negative. No wonder you feel like this! It's your own doing."
"No one ever said life was fair. Just deal with what you've been given."
"There's nothing wrong with you. It's all in your head."
"Stop looking for attention."
"You need to stop feeling sorry for yourself."
"It sounds like you're having another meltdown and going crazy."
"You don't look anxious or depressed. You look fine."

## Juicy Bits

Often, we project our own feelings onto our loved one and assume we know what they need based on what we would need or what we think they "should" need. But this chapter's title is about allowing the person to help us know better how to help them. It gives us a sense of purpose and makes us feel good to be of service. Of course, we must accept that what we can do to help may at times feel small, but it's still valuable.

### Exercise: Listening Practice

It's a common belief that we can't help someone who is going through a mental well-being decline if we aren't a doctor or mental health care professional. But you don't need to be a professional to support someone with their mental health issues. When you communicate and listen non-judgmentally, you *are* helping. So let's practice, and maybe you'll get yourself to a place where you can call yourself a *professional* listener!

1. Plan some of the questions you might ask your loved one to determine what support is needed.

2. Next time you're in a conversation with a friend, colleague, or loved one, pay attention to how much you speak and how much you listen.

3. Practice paraphrasing what you've heard.

## "Will You Hold My Hand for a Little While?"

I came across these beautiful words by Zoe Johansen and felt they encapsulate support in such a profound way. She has given me permission to reprint them here:

*"No need for you to fix anything
No need for you to hold my pain
But will you simply hold my hand?
I do not need your words
Your thoughts
Nor your shoulders to carry me
But will you sit here for a while with me?
Whilst my tears they stream
Whilst my heart it shatters
Whilst my mind plays tricks on me
Will you with your presence let me know that I am not alone, whilst I wander into my inner unknown?
For my darkness is mine to face
My pain is mine to feel
And my wounds are mine to heal
But will you sit with me here, while I courageously show up for it all my dear?
For I am bright because of my darkness
Beautiful because of my brokenness
And strong due to my tender heart
But will you take my hand lovingly, when I sometimes journey into the dark?
I don't ask for you to take my darkness away
I don't expect for you to brighten my day
And I don't believe that you can mend my pain
But I would surely love if you could sit for a while and hold my hand, until I find my way out of my shadowland.
So will you . . . Hold my hand until I return again?"*

Chapter Six

# Handling Unhealthy Behaviors and Setting Boundaries

My mom was a fabulous hostess, full of love and good cheer, and Thanksgiving was an important tradition in our family. But of course, planning and implementing dinner functions for a large family can be stressful, and during higher stress periods, her bipolar symptoms became worse. Sometimes, she had unreasonable expectations, so if something didn't go as planned or wasn't done exactly as she wanted, all hell broke loose.

One particular Thanksgiving in the early 2000s, I found myself in the path of her side effects. To this day, I can't remember the catalyst or the words that were used. I just recall that I could no longer accept the way she was treating me. Survival for my own mental health meant I had to remove myself from the dysfunction.

We didn't speak for another three years.

Mom and I had always been extremely close. Before this incident, we spoke several times a day, and she was a major person in my inner circle. To say the least, leaving that dinner and not speaking for so long was heart-wrenching and challenging.

Looking back, I believe it had to happen. We both needed a breather. If I'd stayed in that unhealthy dynamic, I suspect both of us would have suffered further mental health decline.

When we did come back together, we were stronger, healthier, and more solid than ever. I can't regret setting a boundary and implementing it. I will never accept being on the receiving end of abusive language or poor treatment, just as my mother wouldn't accept that from any of her offspring.

How might things have gone differently? What if I had addressed the behaviors sooner and set boundaries with consequences earlier? Perhaps we wouldn't have missed three years of each other's lives.

In this chapter, let's explore what happens when your own mental health is at risk because of the mental health challenges your loved one faces.

## HOUDINI: THE DISAPPEARING ACT

Have you ever heard the expression, "take your ball and go home"? There have been times in my life when emotions are so heated that the only option seems to be escape. In other words, *get the hell out of Dodge!* That's what I did that day with my mother, and I'm here to tell you that it's okay to do that. It's okay to leave a situation when it risks your own mental well-being.

I'm not suggesting you avoid challenges and sweep anything under the carpet. I'm referring to situations that risk your mental safety. Too often, we think we only have the right to leave if our *physical* safety is at risk, but we also need to safeguard our mental health.

Others may not understand or accept that you left. They might not understand boundaries or the need to protect your own health. Just know that you can love someone and still leave temporarily or even permanently. You can still love them from a distance, whether you're the one who leaves or they're the one who leaves.

Only you know whether you "should" stay or go. I fully get the desire to stay because the other person is in distress. We feel bad for them and pity them, even as we might resent them. But those feelings aren't good for either party.

Of course, remember that people living with mental illness still have the ability to do amazing things. Their disorder doesn't mean they should be pitied for it.

As I've mentioned before, however, the support they receive doesn't always have to come from you. Caring for someone whose behavior is

## Handling Unhealthy Behaviors and Setting Boundaries

detrimental to your own mental health needs to be looked upon as a safety risk.

### Recognizing Abusive Behaviors

As we start to move into setting boundaries, it's key to be aware of abusive behaviors that can impact you mentally, emotionally, and physically. You might have experienced some of these from a loved one without thinking of them as abusive. I invite you to reflect on these behaviors without judgment, as well as the impact they can have on you:

- Blaming you for everything
- Never happy with you, no matter how hard you try or how much you give
- Expecting you to put everything aside to meet their needs
- Making unrealistic or unreasonable demands
- Giving you the silent treatment or withholding affection to punish you when they don't get their way
- Expecting you to agree with them even though you have a different opinion
- Criticizing you for not doing things exactly how they want them done
- Demanding that you devote all your time to them and isolate others
- Gaslighting you by claiming incidents never happened or expecting you to prove that something happened
- Manipulating you into doing things beyond your comfort
- Making fun of you, claiming, "I'm just joking; can't you take a joke?"
- Screaming, shouting, calling you names, and using abusive language when speaking with you
- Refusing to apologize even if you plead and cry, or apologizing repeatedly with no change in behavior

- Damaging your property in angry outbursts, such as throwing objects, punching walls, kicking in doors, etc.
- Physically attacking you, such as pulling your hair, punching, slapping, choking, kicking, or biting you
- Threatening to attack you or threatening to hurt themselves
- Keeping you hostage in your own home or stopping you from calling for help
- Driving recklessly or dangerously when you're in the car with them or telling you to get out of the car on a highway or in an unfamiliar place
- Convincing you to use drugs or alcohol, even if you're in recovery

I've experienced several of the behaviors on this list, so I know how challenging it can be to leave your loved one when they are abusive to you. But it's safest for you and all involved to be physically away from them when you encounter any of these behaviors. There is no excuse for abuse, even though we understand that someone's mental illness can create these behaviors. Regardless of their struggle, you aren't their "punching bag."

When you're safely away from further harm, you can help them find the support they need to assist with their symptoms while you look after your own mental health.

## Impact on Others

When we're dealing with someone's mental health problem or crisis, all eyes tend to be on that person. But their behaviors impact everyone around them. We must not forget about the effects on others in their circle.

Resentment can build when routines and activities are no longer "normal." Other people can be "lost in the shuffle," take "second fiddle" or be put on the "back burner." Please remember to take yourself and others into consideration, too.

## BOUNDARIES

Psychotherapist, relationship expert, and author Terri Cole believes "the act itself of drawing boundaries is communicating clearly about what is okay and what isn't okay with you to the people in your life. It's telling the truth about how you feel and about what you want and need." Terri has written an informative book called *Boundary Boss: The Essential Guide to Talk True, Be Seen, and (Finally) Live Free!* I highly recommend adding this book to your resources.

I've heard others say that boundaries are a form of "tough love." That's true, but I also refer to them as *just love*. Healthy boundaries allow us to love ourselves, as well as others.

Think of snow removal. I have a local snow removal contractor who takes care of my driveway during the winter months. Recently, I was away during the first snowfall of the season, and we got a huge amount of snow. Usually, I'm out there right away shoveling the bits the contractor can't easily access to make sure the boundaries of the driveway are clear. If we don't clear the full path, each time he comes, the path gets narrower until we can barely fit the car in the driveway. When we let snow pile on top of snow, it gets harder and harder to shovel. In some cases, chunks of heavy ice develop that can barely be lifted.

Similarly, by acknowledging, setting, and implementing emotional boundaries earlier, we set up our relationship to be healthier, easing the potential need of repair and the lifting of heavy emotions.

It might seem counterintuitive, but boundaries actually create more freedom, not less. Personally, I find it easier to navigate relationships when people are clear about their boundaries. I'd rather know ahead of time what they consider acceptable behavior. I feel the relationship is more trustworthy, and the boundaries remove the feeling of unease.

Nevertheless, despite all of my training and experience, I still find setting and maintaining boundaries challenging! My people-pleasing ways still win at times. But the harder it is to set a particular boundary, the more likely that boundary needs to be set. In other words, if it's difficult, it's probably very important.

Still, no amount of coaching can put boundaries in place for you. I think about the times I've been in bed, thinking, "Tomorrow, I'll go to the gym." But it doesn't matter unless I actually go to the gym the next day. Boundaries are the same. Talking about them and placing them are two very different things.

Note that boundaries can be physical, emotional, mental, financial, material, or related to time. They can be negotiable or non-negotiable. In order to implement boundaries, you need to first be aware of what behaviors/actions are acceptable to you and which are not. Which ones are you comfortable negotiating, and which ones do you consider to be absolutely non-negotiable?

It's worth mentioning that boundaries aren't about control. Instead, they're meant to express what you're unwilling to accept. Your boundaries are also unique and individual to you. You're allowed to consider a particular behavior unacceptable even if someone else feels differently about it.

The following are some examples of situations that might require boundaries, but this list is not comprehensive. You are allowed to set any boundary that you feel is necessary for your own mental or physical well-being.

- Your loved one's inability to live by agreed rules and consequences in your home
- Disruptive behaviors, such as not coming home at night, playing music too loudly, missing family meals, becoming argumentative
- Showing up at functions intoxicated or high
- How much financial support you are able and willing to provide and how much your loved one contributes to household expenses
- Communication, including its type (text, phone call, etc.) and frequency
- Emotional support limits, knowing when you are at capacity, and setting up other support systems
- Attending support groups
- Going to school/work
- Keeping up with personal hygiene
- Smoking, substance use, alcohol, and/or street drugs in your home

- Gambling and/or gaming limits
- Attending medical appointments, taking prescribed medications

## ACTUALLY SETTING YOUR BOUNDARIES

Involving your loved one in the development of boundaries will encourage a clear understanding between you about what everyone wants, needs, and expects. Discuss and establish basic rules for behavior, cooperation, and limitations. Write them down for clarity's sake.

Of course, if your loved one is unable to participate, boundaries may need to be set without their input. When someone is unwell, aggressive, under the influence of a substance, or unable to think clearly, it's impossible to have a conversation about a broken boundary. We have to enforce the consequences and wait until they have improved before discussing future prevention.

When a boundary is broken, it's imperative that you not excuse their behavior, ignore it, change your mind, or feel guilty for enforcing the consequence. When you don't honor your word and take action, it gives the impression that you aren't committed to the boundary, which essentially cancels it. Even though you might avoid conflict in the moment, you'll have to continue living with the unacceptable behavior. This will only exacerbate your resentment and potentially hurt your relationship with your loved one.

Consequences might include not allowing your loved one in your home, not getting together with them, not providing assistance, not loaning them money, and/or not taking their calls or refusing to continue calls that become abusive.

Others may try to convince you that you're being cruel, but it's important to stick to what you feel is right in the situation. You may want to seek support from outside sources to help you manage and cope.

There's a scene in the 2020 true story film, *Four Good Days*, in which the daughter has a substance use disorder. She shows up at the family home and begs to be let in. The mother (played by Glenn Close) asserts her boundary by not allowing her daughter (played by Mila Kunis) in the house until she's sober. It's heart-wrenching to watch. The daughter ends up sleeping outside on the front porch for days. We see her mother looking out the window, getting very little sleep, and suffering quite an emotional toll. But despite the pain, she stays true to her boundary. Clearly, she loves her daughter and is willing to go to such lengths to support her through healthy boundaries and following through on consequences.

Today, the daughter portrayed in the film is in recovery with the continued support of her mother.

## ASKING VS. DEMANDING

I used to believe that the only way to set boundaries was to demand them. "You do this or else!" I learned otherwise recently when my nephew and nieces came over for a sleepover, and we pitched indoor tents for them. As you can imagine, there were loads of giggles and good times.

As bedtime approached, the kiddies settled into their respective tents. But Linky, my nephew, who always teaches me something, was still up for more fun. He kept the girls awake by tapping on their tent. Eventually, I felt the need to intervene. In a gentle and authoritative voice, I told him to stop bothering the girls and get back in his own tent.

He continued, so I demanded again. When he refused, I could feel my frustration rise. "Linky, for the last time, stop hitting the tent, and get in your own tent. Go to sleep!"

In a matter-of-fact way, he responded, "Not until you say 'please.'" Then he said, "You always expect me to say please, so why don't you?" That hit me hard. Fair enough, Linky.

I said, "Linky, can you PLEASE go in your tent and go to sleep?" He agreed.

When we assert ourselves or set boundaries, we can do it in a confident way that's also loving. We don't have to be aggressive, loud, or demanding. And we can say "please." We can approach in a gentle way, be mindful of our tone, and stay courteous and polite. At the same time, we don't need to over-explain or justify ourselves. We don't have to explain why.

Bear in mind that when you're just starting to set boundaries, you won't be perfect at it. So give yourself some grace. With practice, you'll begin to set boundaries, and no one will even realize you did it!

When we activate a pendulum, it swings fully back and forth until it settles in the middle. When setting boundaries, you may feel you have to take a strong stance at first. But eventually, it will swing into the middle. As each boundary is set, you'll feel more confident about calmly asserting yourself.

## Are You "Enabling"?

People frequently ask me, "How do I know when I'm supporting someone and when I'm enabling them?" Sometimes, what feels like support can actually mean enabling the unhealthy behavior. When we enable, we inadvertently allow someone else's potentially harmful negative patterns, which can slow their progress toward healing.

You may be enabling if you:

- Close your eyes to dangerous behaviors, excessive drinking, and drug misuse
- Fail to hold your loved one accountable for their actions or set boundaries on their behavior
- Partake in the substance use or pick it up and/or pay for it
- Support your loved one financially without addressing the underlying issues that contribute to their mental health problem
- Take care of your loved one's every need, even though they are capable, such as housing, food, car, entertainment, and legal fees
- Avoid conversations about your loved one's mental illness
- Make excuses for a loved one's absence from gatherings, such as in the case of someone with social anxiety, which can encourage avoidance behavior
- Neglect your own needs while making your loved one's needs a priority

In Chapter 3, I wrote that awareness and acknowledgment plus action = change. Do you recognize any of these enabling tendencies in yourself? I know enabling comes from love, so please be gentle with yourself. Remember that awareness is the key to change.

## Enabling Safety First

During a talk I gave at an event, an audience member (I'll call her Susan) told a story about arguing with her adult child (I'll call him Carl) because he wanted to go to a party where there was a risk of using substances and exacerbating the symptoms of his mental health disorder. Carl went to the party anyway, and later that night, he called Susan, asking her to pick him up. On the drive home, he physically attacked his mother. Unfortunately, this was a pattern, and by perpetuating that pattern, Susan was unknowingly enabling her son.

I talked with her about the importance of her own safety. But she felt if she hadn't picked Carl up, he might have harmed himself. Susan was torn between her own safety and that of her son. We talked about the risks to other people as well if she had lost control of the car. So she agreed to put a boundary in place that she wouldn't get in a car with him if he had used a substance or was in the midst of a mental health crisis.

Sometimes, we aren't the best person in the moment to assist our loved one, especially when our own safety is at risk. And our own safety comes first before anyone else's! I know this is extremely difficult, especially when it's our child, but if we allow ourselves to be harmed, we won't be able to *ever* be there for them.

## Guilt over Resentment

An acquaintance of mine gave me permission to share his story in the hope it will be relatable and helpful to those feeling guilty about setting a boundary. Charles and his brother, Jerry, are their only remaining family members. After their mother died, Charles allowed Jerry to temporarily live in his basement until he could get back on his feet after experiencing some mental health challenges. But this arrangement continued for years. In the meantime, Charles was building a career and a family of his own, so his growing family could have used the extra space in the basement. Jerry's mental health symptoms caused him to isolate, not take care of his hygiene, sleep excessively, and play video games constantly. It got to the point that Charles didn't feel free to live his own life fully.

But he felt guilty for no longer wanting his brother to live in the basement. He worried about what would happen to Jerry. At the same time, Charles felt resentful that his brother wasn't taking care of himself. In my support of Charles, I first gave him the opportunity to vent his feelings without fear of judgment. I discussed the importance of boundaries with him in order to protect his own mental health.

Unfortunately, by allowing Jerry to stay, Charles was enabling his brother's behaviors. The situation kept Jerry reliant on Charles and prevented Jerry's growth in his own life. So Charles sat down with his brother, discussed alternatives, and agreed on a timeline. To Charles's surprise, Jerry moved out willingly.

While Jerry still has some challenges today, Charles is able to provide support in a healthier way. He has "a clear mind and heart by setting boundaries and not enabling [Jerry]."

In the book *When the Body Says No: The Cost of Hidden Stress*, author Gabor Maté wrote: "A therapist once said to me, 'If you face the choice between feeling guilt and resentment, choose the guilt every time.' It is wisdom I have passed on to many others since. If a refusal saddles you with guilt, while consent leaves resentment in its wake, opt for the guilt. Resentment is soul suicide." Resentment is also more likely to kill a relationship.

## Capacity vs. Tolerance

In order to determine what you're willing to accept when it comes to the behavior of others, think about your capacity and tolerance levels. It's easy to confuse the two, but they aren't the same. Capacity is what you can manage without causing yourself harm or without too much expense to your well-being. Tolerance is what you can push through and deal with, even if it's at your own mental and/or physical expense. In the chapters that follow, we'll address ways to build your capacity and tolerance.

## Should You Call for Help?

It can be difficult to know when to call for emergency support, an ambulance, police, a doctor, or a crisis line. My rule of thumb is: If the person is at risk of harming themselves or others, are already harmed and/or in need of medical assistance, *make that call.*

Years ago, my partner Dave's dad, Tommy, woke up incoherent and slurring his words. We didn't know if it was his dementia or something else, so we called an ambulance. It turned out that his blood sugar had become dangerously low, putting him extremely close to lapsing into a coma. We got him help just in time.

You may be thinking, "but what if it's nothing?" You might not want to be overly cautious or waste anyone's time. But always err on the side of caution. A first responder in one of my courses said, "We'd rather be called out on a scene and not be needed than not be called and be needed." If you feel the person is in an emergency situation, trust your instincts and CALL, even if it takes some extra courage to do so and even if you think the first responders act as though you have overreacted. Better safe than sorry!

## Tough Decisions

The community worker for my brother, Kevin, called the police when he had a mental health crisis and started to behave erratically. He had stopped taking his medications, and his personal hygiene had been neglected for quite some time. His body was even infested with bed bugs and lice. When my father and I visited him in the hospital, we had to wear head-to-toe protective gear to ensure we didn't become infested ourselves.

Even though Kevin had suffered mental health crises in the past, this felt worse. He was extremely skinny, and they had to shave his head and all the hair off his body to rid him of the bugs. He was in isolation on a locked-down mental health floor.

It was heart-wrenching to see him in this condition. He became frustrated that he couldn't leave the hospital, but the doctors felt strongly that his safety would be at risk if he was released too early. I felt he was in good hands and was confident they had his best interests at heart.

Since he wasn't taking his medication in pill form reliably, they decided to prescribe a medication that would be administered via needle once a month. But he was afraid of needles, so he became angry and combative. "A friend of mine got a needle, and now he limps all the time," Kevin told us.

After several days of refusing his medication, the doctor at the hospital told us we had a choice to make. If Kevin continued to refuse meds, we could sign a form on his behalf that would keep him hospitalized until he was mentally stable and properly medicated. Since I'm well-versed in matters of mental health, our father passed the baton to me as the representative of the family.

Despite my training, it was a very tough decision, so I immediately called other members of our family for their input. I felt in my heart that if I didn't keep my brother in the hospital, his life was in danger. But was I prepared to sign the form, knowing that Kevin would probably be extremely angry with me and might never speak to me again?

I share this story with you because some of you know this feeling all too well. It's horrible to be called to make a difficult decision on behalf of your loved one for their own protection when it goes against their wishes. In my case, I trusted my gut and was prepared to sign the form in the name of love. But I was lucky because just before I had to do it, the doctors convinced Kevin to take his medication.

A few weeks later, they released him to a newly cleaned apartment. He now goes once a month for his "needle," and he's healthy and engaged with life.

Loving someone with a mental health decline can present you with all kinds of difficult scenarios. I often bluntly say, "I'd rather have someone pissed off at me alive than pissed off at me dead."

## Gaslighting

According to the *Merriam-Webster Dictionary*, gaslighting is defined as a "psychological manipulation of a person usually over an extended period of time that causes the victim to question the validity of their own thoughts, perception of reality, or memories and typically leads to confusion, loss of confidence and self-esteem, uncertainty of one's emotional or mental stability, and a dependency on the perpetrator."[1]

In 1944, a film called *Gaslight* portrayed this insidious behavior, including abuse, manipulation, and convincing the victim that what they'd seen had never happened. In my view, "gaslighting" has become a part of pop culture, as more and more people have become aware of it.

We often see it as a symptom of mental illness. The "gaslighter" (yes, I just made it a noun) can keep control of others by effectively denying the reality of their own behavior or its impact. They might deny or minimize their problem, for example, invalidating our concerns. They may distort events to make them seem like no big deal. They may say things like, "You're remembering it wrong; I didn't act that way" or "you must have misunderstood what happened" or "I'm tired of everybody not understanding me" or "I don't have a problem; you're exaggerating." You might be aware they're lying, but they can be so convincing that you start to doubt your own experience.

In my studies to become a body language expert, my teacher and mentor Janine Driver taught me that when someone is lying, they attempt to *convince* us. When someone is truthful, they're more likely to merely try to *convey* what they want to communicate. When you find your loved one trying to convince you of something, it could be an indication that they've resorted to gaslighting.

## Walking on Eggshells

I'm sure you've heard the phrase, "walking on eggshells." It's when a person's unhealthy behaviors cause us to tread carefully around them in an effort to avoid trouble. These behaviors might include angry outbursts, moodiness, or taking offense at what we felt were innocuous statements or actions. So we feel that anything we say or do could set them off.

Many audience members around the world have told me this is how they feel around their loved one who's experiencing a mental well-being decline. They have told me they feel guilty, so they start second-guessing themselves and often come to the conclusion they've done something

---

1. *Merriam-Webster Dictionary*, "Gaslighting," accessed December 20, 2024, https://www.merriam-webster.com/dictionary/gaslighting.

wrong. They feel wobbly, unsure of themselves, and even sometimes sick to their stomach.

If you recognize these feelings, they're red flags that you're experiencing toxic behavior and mistreatment. When you're afraid of upsetting someone all the time, it severely affects your nervous system. I will discuss this topic further, but just know that when you feel like you're walking on eggshells, it's an important moment for self-care and setting boundaries. As the Dalai Lama has said, "Don't let the behavior of others destroy your inner peace."

## "You Made Me"

As I mentioned, it's a common occurrence for people experiencing a mental health problem or crisis to blame others for what's happening. Their feelings can be so overwhelming that they project onto others, and by doing so, they avoid not taking responsibility for their own actions. Sometimes, it's blatantly obvious, and you know unequivocally that you're not to blame. Other times, you might find yourself believing that it was your responsibility.

I had an "aha" moment when I was taking care of my nephew, Linky. When it was time for bed, I told everyone to put on their jammies. As most kids do, he started to make excuses to stall. "I'm thirsty. Can I have some milk?"

I responded, "Sure. After you put on your jammies, I'll get you some milk." This became a standoff. He was determined to get his milk immediately! In an effort to persuade me, he dramatically fell off of his chair (no kids were harmed) and said, crying, "Look what you made me do!"

I was nowhere near him. He chose to "fall" off the chair. I calmly explained this to him and gave him milk while we sat at the table. It was then a great opportunity to discuss with him that these kinds of interactions aren't good for either of us and that we needed to do it differently in the future. He put on his jammies, and we had a peaceful goodnight cuddle.

Although the above scenario is somewhat typical of a child's behavior, it reminded me that nobody can "make us" do anything. There's always a choice. Yes, there are factors that contribute to behaviors, but we aren't responsible for the actions of others. I'm going to say it again: YOU are not responsible for your loved one's choices or actions.

## When Tempers Rise

It isn't unusual for tempers to flare when people become angry and emotional. It's important to do your best to prevent a situation from escalating, which risks harm for all involved.

For example, my twin brother owns a security guard agency, and they patrol an area where many individuals with mental health issues tend to hang out. It isn't uncommon for him to be in a position to de-escalate tense situations. In fact, he trains his staff in these kinds of techniques and the proper use of force vs. the improper use of force. Along with using some of the tools I recommended in Chapters 4 and 5, he suggests the following evidence-based strategies, which have been successful in managing individuals who are in distress:

- Always respect their personal space, give the person room to move, and allow them to walk up and down if need be. Keep an appropriate distance to prevent them from feeling threatened or overwhelmed. An audience member once shared with me that when a situation starts to escalate in their family, they say their code word, and everyone backs off. They give the person space and the chance to get some fresh air before continuing the conversation more calmly.
- Approach with a calm, relaxed posture, and be mindful to keep your tone of voice gentle rather than firm or authoritative.
- Take care not to overreact or escalate your emotions. This helps to create a stable environment that will assist the person in calming down.
- It's important to stay focused on the issue at hand in order to keep the discussion productive and avoid arguments.
- Set clear, consistent boundaries, and communicate these calmly and assertively. This clarity helps prevent misunderstandings and establishes a framework for positive interactions.

- Prioritize what's most important, and let go of less critical issues. Focus solely on resolving the issue at hand as effectively as possible.
- Silence is golden. Pausing can give both parties a chance to reflect and process what has been said, allowing for emotions to settle.
- Allow time for decisions to be made. This shows respect for the person's autonomy and can lead to better outcomes. When people feel they have been heard and that they matter, they're more likely to respond positively.

*Regardless of the content of this chapter, please note that people living with mental illness are rarely the aggressor. In fact, they're more likely to be the victim of those who fear them. Others may believe they need to defend themselves and/ or attack due to a false belief that people with mental health issues are dangerous.*

## Juicy Bits

Your safety is always the priority. When you're faced with a physically dangerous or emotionally charged situation or environment, the best course of action is often to take your ball and go home. This isn't an avoidance tactic. It's self-preservation and self-care. And yes, it's tough love toward the other person.

It's important to face the fact that when it gets to a certain point, you won't be able to win an argument with someone in a mental health crisis. Subjecting yourself to abusive behavior is a risk to your own mental health. It's also important to remember that their behaviors don't define who they are. My mother used to say, "I don't want to do these things, but I can't stop myself."

Only you can determine if you "should" stay or go, but I urge you to choose your own mental health more often than I suspect you're currently doing. You might have great compassion for your loved one, but that doesn't mean you have to subject yourself to physical or emotional harm. The situation also doesn't have to be explosive to be harmful to you. Outbursts can be passive, and the silent treatment can be very loud. Whatever you do, set boundaries to protect yourself. As the adage goes, "Don't light yourself on fire so they can be warm."

## EXERCISE: SELF-CARE AND BOUNDARIES

Setting and implementing boundaries is vital for handling unhealthy behaviors, but bear in mind that someone with a mental health disorder may challenge those boundaries. This will require courage, patience, repetition, and resilience on your part. Go with grace and compassion for everyone involved, including yourself!

Here are some ways you can prepare for the situations discussed in this chapter:

1. Write about what came up for you while reading the chapter.

2. Make a list of how you may have enabled your loved one(s).

3. I invite you to take into consideration and write down the benefits for you of enabling your loved one's behaviors. Maybe you haven't put a boundary in place in order to "keep the peace," or it makes you feel good to help. Perhaps you're sure if you do this, it will help them get better so that they'll no longer need you. Don't judge yourself. Under challenging circumstances, you've done the best you knew how.

4. Write down your desired boundaries, including what you're willing to accept and not willing to accept.

5. Pick one boundary, and write down what you will say to your loved one when you set it. Practice saying it out loud.

Chapter Seven

# Avoiding Burnout

As I started to write this chapter, I thought I'd practice what I preach. So I decided to go outside and clean up the fresh snow as an act of self-care. I find shoveling light snow, making snow angels, and breathing in the fresh air to be a great opportunity for pause and rejuvenation.

It was a cold day, but since I didn't think I'd be outside long, I didn't wear a scarf or socks. I also didn't take my keys, thinking I'd just go back in through the garage.

I was outside for about forty-five minutes when I started to feel cold. I punched in the garage code, but to my surprise, the door wouldn't open.

There I was, feeling cold as it started to get dark, and I had no means of getting into my house. I tried the code several times to no avail. Thank goodness I had my cellphone with me, so I called my partner, Dave, who was more than an hour's drive away.

"I've gotten myself in a bit of a predicament," I told him. I still hadn't fully realized the severity of the situation. We troubleshooted the problem, and I searched the internet on my phone for solutions. I had gone out without my glasses, however, so everything looked blurry.

Dave suggested I take the twenty-minute walk to the local restaurant to keep warm until he arrived, but without socks or proper snow boots, I could slip or get frostbitten toes!

Plan B was to seek a neighbor's help, which felt awkward and uncomfortable. But as time ticked by, and I felt colder, I was left with no other option. Thankfully, a neighbor came over and discovered that the battery in my garage door remote was low. He had just the right battery, and voila! I could get inside. I was so grateful for his help and for the warmth and safety of my home.

Years ago, this situation would have spun me into a panic. I would have succumbed to worst-case scenario thinking to the point of "freezing" my brain so that I couldn't think my way out. I probably would have beaten myself up about it, thinking to myself, "How could you go outside without the proper gear or keys?"

But this time, I was able to focus on the task at hand. I've learned to invest my energy in what I can control, focus on what needs to happen in the moment, and learn from the experience for the next time. I noticed symbolism in my experience, however, because burnout can feel like being trapped outside with no apparent way to get back in.

Before burnout strikes, most of us are aware of our high stress level, but it can still feel like it comes out of nowhere. All of a sudden, we're no longer equipped to manage the basics.

In my snow situation, I was caught off guard and ill-prepared. I didn't ensure I had the tools to keep warm if something didn't go as planned. This chapter is designed to make sure you aren't caught off guard and ill-prepared for burnout.

So let's dive into some of the causes, signs, and symptoms of burnout and how you can equip yourself with the tools of self-care while navigating your loved one's mental well-being decline.

## Causes of Burnout

The term *burnout* was coined by psychologist Herbert J. Freudenberger in the 1970s. He believed that those of us who are prone to it are dedicated and committed. He wrote: "It is precisely because we are dedicated that we walk into a burn-out trap. We feel a pressure from within to work and help and we feel a pressure from the outside to give."[1] But burnout can lead to severe stress that results in extreme physical, mental, and/or emotional exhaustion.

As we've seen, loving someone who's going through a mental well-being decline can be challenging. When these challenges exceed our

---

1. Herbert J. Freudenberger, "Staff Burn-Out," *Journal of Social Issues*, Winter 1974, accessed January 15, 2025, https://doi.org/10.1111/j.1540-4560.1974.tb00706.x.

ability to cope, we experience emotional and physical turmoil, resulting in what some refer to as "caregiver burnout." But we don't have to be someone's caregiver to experience burnout. Loving the person and being around them while they're suffering can be enough to put us at risk.

Some of the causes of burnout include:

- Overcommitting
- Overextending
- Lack of boundaries
- Saying "yes" excessively and rarely saying "no" to requests
- Overworking
- Lack of supportive friends and professional help
- A toxic home environment
- Lack of sufficient resources
- Lack of self-care
- Lack of a feeling of purpose

## SIGNS AND SYMPTOMS OF BURNOUT

*Feeling overwhelmed, exhausted, and depleted physically and emotionally.* We may isolate, no longer socializing and confiding in friends, family members, and coworkers. Physical symptoms may include headaches, nervous stomach, or stomach aches.

*Easily getting sick.* Burnout can weaken our immune system, making us more susceptible to colds, flu, and other viruses.

*Stress-related symptoms.* Burnout can lead to brain fog, anxiety, or depression.

*Numbing out or "daydreaming."* We may dream about running away or "getting away from it all" on a vacation. We might look for ways to numb our emotional pain with drugs, alcohol, and/or food.

*Changes in appetite or sleep patterns.* We might sleep too much, too little, or not be able to get to sleep.

*Easily irritated.* It isn't uncommon when we're burned out to be short with friends, coworkers, and family members. Coping with day-to-day stressors or tasks may start to feel impossible, especially when things don't go as planned.

*Hopelessness/helplessness.* We might feel apathetic and empty, saying "what's the point?"

## SELF-CARE TO WARD OFF BURNOUT

According to the National Institute of Mental Health: "Self-care means taking the time to do things that help you live well and improve both your physical health and mental health. This can help you manage stress, lower your risk of illness, and increase your energy. Even small acts of self-care in your daily life can have a big impact."[2]

Self-care can be instrumental in warding off burnout and maintaining or improving your mental health. It's a must for self-preservation regardless of the challenges we face. It's also a "workout" for building resilience, which we'll talk about in more detail in the next chapter.

It's important *not* to think of self-care as a reward, however. We don't have to "earn" it, justify it, or defend it. We *need* it, and we're worthy of it by the mere fact that we're human. So I encourage you to add some form of self-care daily.

You may be thinking, "but, Yvette, isn't it selfish to think of myself, especially when my loved one needs me more?" When someone is selfish, it's because they're doing things for themselves to the detriment of others. Self-care is doing things for yourself for the *betterment* of others, as well as yourself. It makes you more equipped to be helpful to others. It's a win-win! In fact, our loved ones actually need us to pay attention to self-care. *Read that again!* We forget it all too often, but we can't give our best to others unless we first take care of ourselves.

How often do we wait until we're fully sick before we give ourselves any downtime? Why do we tend to wait until we can't function *before* we give ourselves rest, relaxation, and rejuvenation? I'm sure you've heard the sayings, "you can't serve from an empty cup" or "you can't drive a car on an empty tank."

---

2. National Institute of Mental Health, "Caring for Your Mental Health," last updated December 2024, accessed January 15, 2025, https://www.nimh.nih.gov/health/topics/caring-for-your-mental-health#:~:text=Self%2Dcare%20means%20taking%20the,can%20have%20a%20big%20impact.

A massage therapist recently said to me, "People deserve a massage like this." I asked her how often she gives herself the gift of a massage. She said she loves giving massages, but she doesn't receive them. We spoke about including herself in the picture. How often do you take care of everyone else, but when it comes to yourself, you make excuses? I invite you to make sure you get back as much as you give.

Actress Jamie Lee Curtis once said, "Hurt people hurt people; I also think you can add to that, helped people help people."

## Bringing Back the **SELF**

To be the best version of yourself and avoid burnout, the most powerful thing you can do is include yourSELF in the picture.

Not long ago, I got a call from a loved one looking for support with a significant other who was going through a mental well-being decline. The spouse's behaviors were directly affecting both of them. After listening non-judgmentally, I helped them understand the next step for them: "be in care of yourSELF."

Start with the SELF. What are YOU feeling? How are YOU managing YOUR feelings? How is this situation impacting YOU? What support do YOU need? How can YOU be in care of YOURSELF?

Again, I know this is counterintuitive. It isn't what we're taught to do. And if others around you aren't used to it, you might ruffle some feathers! As I mentioned earlier, I have heard statements like, "must be nice you have time for that" or "must be nice you can afford that."

I encourage you to practice self-care anyway, despite any naysayers. When I saw the difference it made in my mental/physical health, home life, business, and relationships, I realized I could no longer afford to live without it. People around me started to notice the significance of self-care for themselves and said things like, "I'll have what she's having" and "I think she's onto something! Me, too, please."

I understood firsthand the importance of self-care when my psychotherapy training program included personal therapy. In the Mental Health First Aid course I facilitate, they even added "S" in their acronym of actions for self-care for the first aider! That's how important it is.

## Self-Care Is Unique to You

I often go to the Nordik spa because there are proven physical and mental benefits to cycling our body through hot water followed by cold water and a period of rest. But contrary to popular belief, self-care isn't all about spa days and bubble baths. We are all unique in terms of the types of self-care we prefer.

For example, have you ever seen a bag of multicolored popcorn kernels? Although the various colored kernels have the same cooking process, they pop at varying degrees, and when they pop, they all turn into fluffy white popcorn. All the colors still have the same result. Whatever the type of self-care you choose, it will benefit you by healing your burnout, building resilience, and rejuvenating you.

Self-care can involve something as simple as giving yourself what I call a "coffee facial" as the steam rises out of the coffeemaker. Try hovering your face over it, and inhale the freshly steamed coffee smell.

Self-care can be celebrating the "small" things. Perhaps a few outwardly vocal cheers when you get in the car and realize your partner filled your tank with gas, saving you a trip to the station.

Self-care can be visualizing what a perfect day might look like for you. Are you on a boat with the sun shining down or snuggled on the couch in your jammies watching your favorite TV series?

Self-care can be walking your pets, blowing bubbles, acting like a kid again, bouncing a ball, playing with a coloring book, taking up a hobby, jumping in a pile of leaves, dressing up for Halloween, decorating the house for a special occasion, or dancing, even if you think you look foolish! Do anything that brings you joy or peace.

Self-care can even involve decluttering your home. I used to keep a cluttered space because my mental health tended to be scattered. This often created frustration and stress for me because I couldn't find things. Plus, just the sight of a messy space was demoralizing, making me feel overwhelmed and unmotivated to do anything.

Self-care can be hiring someone to help you declutter. Motivational speaker Jack Canfield often speaks about hiring someone to do the things we don't want to do. This frees us up to do the things we *do* want to do. As a result, we have more energy, less stress, and better mental health. I understand that not everyone can afford this, but it might be possible to spend less on something that isn't as supportive and more on your self-care instead.

Of course, self-care also sometimes means doing things we don't necessarily "want" to do, such as going to doctors, the dentist, exercising, eating healthy, or creating a budget. These are good for us, even if they aren't always fun.

Sometimes, it means pushing the limits for our peace of mind. For example, a while back, my company secured a big contract for facilitating courses on mental health. Just before the first course, I became ill. I did my best to be ready for the event, but I woke up that morning unsure how I could do it. I debated canceling. But the idea of that caused me such stress that I decided to muster up all of my energy and show up. Otherwise, I would have catastrophized and worried about how canceling would affect my future. So I took care of my mental health by going forward with the event and immediately took care of my physical health afterward. As the saying goes, "the show must go on," and despite not feeling my best, I got rave reviews. In another situation, of course, I might have felt it was best to cancel.

We have to make decisions based on our specific circumstances. Again, self-care is unique and very personal. Always give yourself permission to do it your way, and use your intuition to determine what works best for you.

There are no quick fixes, however. Self-care is a lifetime process, not a one-and-done kind of thing. You don't brush your teeth once and then never again! But since we aren't taught self-care beyond basic hygiene, we have to make more of an effort to do it. I continue to need reminders to put self-care into practice on a regular basis.

## SELF-CARE MYTHS

There are no rules to self-care, and even if we do take excellent care of ourselves, we will still experience some stress. That's just life.

How often do we blame ourselves when we become ill or go through a challenging time? We think, "if only I had done _____, this wouldn't have happened." But self-care doesn't necessarily prevent negative experiences. What it does is make us better equipped to handle the challenges that come our way. (We'll talk more about resilience in the next chapter.)

Be careful, too, not to make self-care a chore that you "have" to do. Then it becomes its own stressor, which is the opposite of what it's intended to be. You might, for example, tell yourself that self-care means unplugging from communications and putting your cellphone on silent. I once visited a spa with a few friends, and I needed to keep my finger on the pulse of my business. So I would go to the locker room and periodically check my cellphone. My friends said, "You're at a spa! You're supposed to take a break from that!" I didn't check my messages as often as I normally would, but I knew it would stress me out more if I didn't check them at all. For me, it was a form of self-care to check periodically. That way, I could enjoy my quiet time, knowing all was well with my business.

It's also important to acknowledge that there's no fail-proof form of self-care. Perhaps what worked for you before won't work for you at another time. Think of it as "inspired action." Some people might like to put self-care on their to-do list, but I prefer to be inspired. There's no right or wrong way to do it. The point is that it helps you. If it doesn't, try something else.

A few years ago, walking was a form of my self-care for both my physical and mental health. I put it on a daily to-do list and had a goal of up to four kilometers a day. At the time, I needed to set that expectation for myself to encourage me to fit it into my schedule no matter what. It was great for a couple of months, and I benefited from the improvements it provided. Then one day, my leg cramped up, and I had to find the nearest pole to lean on and stretch it out. I soon found out I had sciatica caused by a degenerative disc disease that created debilitating nerve pain from my lower back all the way down to my toes. At times, I had to practically crawl up the stairs to bed or be escorted in a wheelchair, and I needed a cane to keep my balance. It was sixteen weeks of hell! Walking wasn't an option until I healed, so I had to shift my forms of self-care.

When I was able to walk again, I stopped putting it on my to-do list. Instead, I walked because I COULD! I walked as far or as short a distance as I felt inspired to go.

Self-care also doesn't have to be all or nothing. Always look for the thing you CAN do, and do the best you can with the energy you have. Can't clean your room? Clean a corner of it. Can't make your bed? Throw a blanket over it. Can't do all the dishes? Do one dish. Can't brush your teeth? Rinse with mouthwash. Can't put makeup on? Wash your face. One percent beats 0 percent every time! You may be surprised to discover that giving 1 percent provides you with the energy to then give 2 percent, 5 percent, 10 percent, or even more! Try one small act of self-care, and don't judge it if that's all you can manage that day. Just make sure that you don't give so much energy to others that you have nothing left for yourself. That's when you'll need to shift how you spend your energy.

Self-care involves allowing others to be in care of you as well! When I couldn't walk, I had no choice but to allow others to support me. I had to put my ego aside and accept the help.

## Managing Your Expectations

Managing my expectations of myself and others has proven to be an important aspect of self-care, especially in avoiding burnout. In the past, I spent too much time trying to be perfect, while worrying what others thought about me.

The National Library of Medicine shares Jeannette Y. Wick's view that managing expectations means communicating to make sure everyone involved has a clear understanding of what to expect, as well as when to expect it.[3]

When I'm about to do something that causes me anxiety, I look at how I can best manage my expectations. For example, driving in a foreign country on the opposite side of the road and navigating roundabouts are extremely stressful for me. To avoid any mishaps, I reflect on the support I need. A few years ago, I was the designated driver while visiting relatives in the UK with my dad as my passenger and co-pilot. I asked him to do his best to avoid gasps or frightened facial expressions when I didn't drive perfectly. When we came to a roundabout, I asked him to

---

3. J. Y. Wick, "Managing Expectations: 'What Do You Mean?'", *Consultant Pharmacist* 28, no. 1 (2013), 58–62, doi:10.4140/TCP.n.2013.58.

navigate the road signs and guide me to the proper lane so that I could solely focus on the fast cars around me. This helped me stay calmer. I also requested that he not panic if I missed a roundabout turn, which might require retracing our steps.

My dad was so supportive that he did all of that and more. He encouraged me by saying, "keep up the great work!" And he maintained a great sense of humor throughout.

Fast forward a few years later, we were in Northern Ireland, where we had to navigate roundabouts again. Along with managing expectations, I added staying mindful of how I spoke to myself during the drives. I also gave myself pep talks leading up to the trip. With my previous foreign country driving experience, my self-care tools in place, managing expectations, communicating the kind of support I needed, and my pep talk prior to the trip, I drove like a champ! I navigated narrow roads with bushes and cars zooming inches away from us. Although it was still scary at times, I gave myself permission not to be perfect.

Also allow the situation to be less than perfect. I learned this on an Alaska trip with Dave. We were about to go on an excursion to the Ketchikan rainforest sanctuary on an extremely rainy day. To get there, we had to take a boat ride on a rigid-hull inflatable—an open motorized ocean raft called a Seahawk. Some refer to it as "banana boat." They provided outdoor gear to keep us comfortable in the rain, but there wasn't enough for everyone. The tour guide said something so profound that it has stuck with me: "You are going to get wet; no amount of gear is going to keep you dry." The comment changed my perspective and helped me manage my expectations. As a result, I released the need to be protected from the rain and embraced the journey, even if I got wet.

When you are navigating yourself through a loved one's mental well-being decline, you ARE going to get "wet." You're likely to feel angry, disappointed, confused, guilty, sad, frustrated, apathetic, desperate, and more. Rather than focusing on trying to control the circumstances or avoid your feelings, manage your expectations while embracing what is.

How can you best prepare by managing your expectations when supporting your loved one through a mental well-being decline? Are you expecting too much from yourself, from them, or from others?

## CREATE A SAFE SPACE

Creating a safe space where you can find solace, recharge, and reconnect with yourself is essential for your mental and emotional well-being. You may have heard the terms *man cave* or *girl pad*. These are great, but you can also simply create an altar at home for spiritual practice that can give you solace.

A sacred space for your chosen form of self-care can be instrumental in managing your stress. It's your safe haven where you can be yourself, express your thoughts and emotions, and engage in self-care activities without distractions or fear of judgment. So it needs to be a place where you feel comfortable and secure.

When choosing your safe space, ensure that it's private and with limited interruptions. Create a peaceful, decluttered environment. Make it calming with lower lighting and perhaps some essential oils or incense. There are some great essential oils that support positive mental health, such as lavender, rose, chamomile, frankincense, lemon, bergamot, and peppermint. Decorate the space with items that make you feel good, such as photos, artwork, or objects that are of special significance to you. It doesn't have to be a big space. It can simply be a chair or a small table area. Just make sure it's peaceful.

## HARP ON HAPPY

Recently, I saw a video on Instagram by Molly Scullion in which she acknowledged all the extra stressors that went along with planning a wedding. She refused to get bogged down by her to-do list. Instead, she encouraged herself and others to "harp on happy." After all, she was getting to have a wedding and be married to the man she loved!

When you think of what makes you feel good, it will help you better manage your stressors. Molly's attitude shift helped me change the way I felt about my book deadline! I was putting all kinds of extra deadlines on myself. At times, I had to drag myself to the computer to write, feeling weighed down by the pressure. It was a game-changer when I shifted my thoughts to "I GET to write a book!" I'm happy for the opportunity to be of service and share my knowledge and experience with others. This overrides the pressure.

Are you giving yourself permission to feel happy in the face of your challenges? What brings you joy? I invite you to *harp on happy*.

## It's a Laughing Matter

Laughter is a great stress reliever, even if we're forcing it. It's almost impossible to feel anxious, angry, or sad when we're laughing. A good old-fashioned belly laugh revs up and then cools down our stress response. It helps us relax, reduce stress, and increase our energy. It can even increase and then decrease our heart rate and blood pressure, leaving us with a good, tranquil feeling.

Laughter can make it easier to cope with difficult situations and help us connect with other people. It helps us put things in perspective and provides the psychological space to navigate conflict and overwhelming feelings.

It's also contagious. When someone else starts laughing, it's hard for us not to join in. Laughter among friends, family, or work colleagues can have a profound effect on all aspects of our mental and emotional health. So I encourage you to bring more laughter into your own life. Humor is a great and healthy coping mechanism.

In fact, make it a habit to spend time with friends who make you laugh. That can be a wonderful addition to your self-care routine. If you have inside jokes with friends, it can be a great stress reliever. Maybe it's a certain look or a head nod that always evokes laughter.

You might even consider trying laughter yoga that gets people laughing together. Or go to a comedy or improv show. If you tend to choose drama or action movies, try some comedies instead!

Of course, please be mindful not to laugh at the expense of others. My family has always found bathroom humor hilarious, for example, but it's considered inappropriate in some circles. I also used to be self-deprecating to be funny, but then I realized I was putting myself down. So as you seek out more laughter in your life, be careful to discern a good joke from a bad or hurtful one.

## Decluttering the Mind

The American Psychological Association describes mindfulness as an "awareness of one's internal states and surroundings. Mindfulness can help people avoid destructive or automatic habits and responses by learning to observe their thoughts, emotions, and other present-moment experiences without judging or reacting to them."[4]

Some of the benefits of mindfulness include less emotional reactivity, the ability to focus, more cognitive flexibility, and better relationship satisfaction.

Meditation is a popular mindfulness technique that has been around for thousands of years. It has proven to help people manage stress by grounding them in the present. Meditation doesn't have to mean sitting still with music or in complete silence. It can be anything that reduces the chatter in the mind, such as focusing on something repetitive like knitting, gardening, or going for a walk.

Some of the emotional benefits of meditation include more self-awareness, improved patience, a different perspective on life challenges, and a reduction of negative feelings. Over the years, I have become more and more aware of how much noise is in my head. Are you aware of the noise in your own mind? The good news is that mindfulness helps us become more adept at choosing the noise we want to relinquish versus the thoughts we want to keep.

When going through a loved one's mental well-being decline, it helps to have a calmer mind. One of the ways we do this is by decluttering the noise. Lately, I've focused on the technology that keeps my mind cluttered. Do I really need to answer that text right away, or can I set aside a better time to respond? How about that inbox full of emails that are no longer necessary? How about deleting and unsubscribing from emails that no longer serve us? While writing this book, I discovered how distracted and cluttered my mind can get. Now, I often turn on the phone's Do Not Disturb mode to keep my mind focused.

Here's another tip: remember your five senses. One of the fastest ways to come back to the present moment and disengage from the mind's chatter is to "stop and smell the roses." Literally! Go outside, take a deep breath, and take in the environment. What does it smell and feel like? Feel the breath move into your belly, and then exhale deeply.

---

4. American Psychological Association, "Mindfulness," accessed January 17, 2025, https://www.apa.org/topics/mindfulness.

Paying attention to your senses will take you back to simpler times. I know it may sound trivial, but connecting to your senses and happy memories can provide a fresh perspective and do wonders to help you alleviate stress.

## DOING NOTHING IS SOMETHING

I'm a doer—a type "A" personality who is usually on the go. I tend to jump right into action and fix-it mode, so I have to consciously make time to pause. It isn't easy, but I'm always grateful when I take that time. When navigating ourselves though a loved one's mental well-being decline, we're often in situations we can't control. And it sometimes feels as though none of our self-care tools are working. We feel at a loss as to what to do, throwing our hands in the air.

This isn't necessarily a bad thing. Taking our hands off of our perceived controls and pausing is an opportunity to be aware of our emotions and default settings. It also gives space for our loved one to empower themselves without us rushing to try to fix them.

Pausing may look like a "duvet day," as my Aunty Eileen calls it. This means staying in bed under the covers or diving your nose deep into a book. It could mean getting out into nature, feeling the breeze on your face, and smelling the fresh air. Pausing may mean taking a cat nap. (Always remember that rest is productive!)

Pausing might mean choosing not to give advice in order to genuinely listen and be fully present with the other person. It may mean allowing your emotions to surface and giving yourself space to feel them.

In a pause, we discontinue whatever we've been doing, thinking, planning, and worrying about. We become fully present, attentive, and still. We just *stop*, allowing the chips to fall where they may.

When we get out of our own way, pause, and stop *doing*, we can focus on *being*. Then we may notice that some situations resolve themselves. Sometimes, doing nothing *is* doing something.

## FOCUS ON THE TASK AT HAND

When my mom was diagnosed with cancer in 2011, it happened to be at the same time I was transitioning between homes. Instead of moving into my new place, I opted to move all of my belongings into storage so that I could move back to the family home and support my parents. I lived with them for six months, along with my cats.

After my mom recovered from surgery, I was in the midst of planning my move back north when my cat, Tava, became ill. On my mother's birthday, while giving my cat a belly rub, I found a lump. The symbolism wasn't lost on me. My mother's lump had been removed, but suddenly, Tava had a lump, too. Even though I was days away from moving, I knew I had to take Tava to the vet.

As I was leaving for the vet with Tava's cat fur stuck to my wet, sobbing face, I shared my anxiety and panic with my dad. "What if it's cancer? What if she doesn't come home from the vet? What if my other cat can't live without her? What if I can't move back north?"

My dad listened patiently and then said, "Yvette, focus on the task at hand." The task was to get Tava to the vet, which was all I could control in that moment. That's all I had to think about during the car ride. I put all other thoughts and worries on the back burner. I even visualized putting them in a box with a lock. I could always go back to those thoughts and deal with them later. Any time another worry surfaced, I told myself "not now." It brought me enormous comfort.

As you can imagine, it was a very challenging day. Sadly, I had to leave Tava behind. She was very sick, and there was nothing more we could do for her. I got through the day by literally focusing on each task at hand. The next task was celebrating my mom's birthday. I was emotional about Tava, but I didn't want to miss that special occasion, especially after my mom had battled cancer.

Since that day, anytime I find myself speculating about "what ifs," I remember my dad's advice. Focusing on the task at hand has proven to be the best sage advice I've received to date, and I love that it came from my father! I use it frequently, and on many occasions, it has been "first aid" for my mental health. I invite you to try this the next time you get caught up in the what ifs and risk burnout. Focus on the one thing you can do in that moment. Maybe it's listening, getting help, decluttering your mind, or doing one small act of self-care.

## Seeking Therapy

You may be experiencing a temporary problem that can be helped with supportive family, friends, and your own "toolbox." But at times, you might need professional support for the challenges you're facing. If you're experiencing ongoing distress or stress that's interfering with your life in any of the following ways, it may be time to see a therapist:

- The quality of your life has decreased significantly or is decreasing
- Your daily activities, school, work, or relationships are negatively impacted
- You feel controlled by your symptoms
- There's a risk of harm to yourself or others
- You feel overwhelmed or tired all the time
- You feel a disproportionate amount of anger, rage, or resentment
- You feel anxious or panicky
- You feel apathetic or hopeless
- You feel shame and have withdrawn socially

Depending on what you're experiencing, there are many types of therapy available. Sometimes, I need support physically, so I might seek a naturopath, massage therapist, acupuncturist, osteopath, etc. These, in turn, will help my mental health.

The connection between the mind and body never ceases to amaze me. When something manifests physically, it can create a risk to our mental health, and when the mind experiences symptoms, it can directly impact us physically.

Here are a few different approaches to therapy:

*Psychodynamic therapy* is based on the principles of psychoanalysis and is an in-depth form of "talk therapy." It involves recognizing, acknowledging, and overcoming negative feelings and repressed emotions to improve our relationship with ourselves, with others, and with the world around us.

*Behavioral therapy* emphasizes that certain destructive behaviors develop from what we learned in our past, and this technique can help us change those behaviors.

*Cognitive behavioral therapy (CBT)* is another form of behavioral therapy that's often used to treat mental health conditions and substance use disorders. It focuses on the connection between thoughts, feelings, and behaviors.

*Integrative or holistic therapy* considers the whole person—mind, body, and spirit.

Any of these modalities can be a wonderful complement to conventional treatments. Within the above-mentioned categories, there are a variety of more specialized approaches that you can explore.

## ONE SIZE DOESN'T FIT ALL

You may need to see more than one therapist before you find the one who is right for you. After a few sessions with my very first therapist, there wasn't much progress. They were lovely, empathetic, and provided a safe space for me. But I needed someone who would challenge me, go deeper, and help me grow and heal. Working with my next therapist provided the opportunity for me to do just that. Letting my previous therapist know that I didn't think we were a fit was challenging, but it allowed me to speak my truth. I grew stronger as a result. I believe there are no "waste of time" therapeutic experiences, but therapists are all as individual and unique as the rest of us.

Therapy gave me the ability to heal, grow, and be of service to others while being in care of myself. It wasn't always easy, but it was worth it every step of the way! As Brené Brown says, "Truth and courage aren't always comfortable, but they are never weakness."

## INCREASE YOUR DOPAMINE

The Cleveland Clinic describes dopamine as "a neurotransmitter made in your brain. It plays a role as a 'reward center' and in many body functions, including memory, movement, motivation, mood, attention and more. As a hormone, dopamine is released into your bloodstream. It plays a small role in the 'fight-or-flight' syndrome. The fight-or-flight response refers to your body's response to a perceived or real stressful situation, such as needing to escape danger."[5] Experts believe that having enough dopamine in our body helps us feel happier, more motivated, more alert, and more focused. So how do we get some more of that "feel-good" hormone in a natural, healthy way?

Research shows that exercise can improve mood and raise dopamine levels, as well as endorphin levels (another feel-good hormone). Meditating and/or listening to music is another good way to stimulate a dopamine release in the brain.

The sun's ultraviolet rays help us produce dopamine (along with vitamin D), which is vital for our mental health. (During winter, we might feel the impact of getting less sunlight.)

I'll talk more about food in the next chapter, but studies show that eating protein can help boost dopamine levels as well.

## Scream It Out

Screaming can be used as a therapeutic tool. It's referred to as scream therapy or primal therapy and was developed in the 1970s by psychologist Arthur Janov. Screaming helps release pent-up emotions, frustrations, and psychological pain. The concept is that when we scream, it acts as a release valve to blow off steam.

Screaming is also an ancient form of Chinese medicine that has been passed on from generation to generation. They believe yelling is good exercise for our lungs and liver.

I recommend giving it a go by screaming into your pillow, in your car, or in your bathroom. If you plan on screaming outside or around other people, however, it might be a good idea to forewarn them!

## Gratitude Journal

No matter what's happening, there's always something to be grateful for. I feel grateful for my breath, warmth, the ability to walk and see, and

---

5. Cleveland Clinic, "Dopamine," last reviewed March 23, 2022, accessed January 17, 2025, https://my.clevelandclinic.org/health/articles/22581-dopamine.

my bed. Being grateful for waking up reminds me of my Auntie Tish, whom we lost to cancer a few years back. When I went to visit her on her deathbed, she said, "When I wake up, I give thanks that I didn't wake up dead!" It's a funny statement, yet so profound.

Perhaps you might be grateful for what has brought you to this moment. Every one of us has gone through hardships that led us to this time and place. As I have mentioned before, sometimes we need to remind ourselves of what helped us in the past, which could also help us now. What resources or people did you rely on at that time? What skills did you develop, such as resilience, persistence, determination, grace, or patience?

Keeping a journal is beneficial for your mental health. I recommend writing down in your journal what you're grateful for. You might even want to adopt this as a daily practice to help you come back to the present moment and appreciate what you *do* have.

## Juicy Bits

Some people may think burnout is inevitable when we deal regularly with people in mental health decline, but it doesn't have to be. If we know what to do to take proper care of ourselves, we can often head it off at the pass.

And let's change the narrative from thinking of self-care as selfish or as a luxury, and let's stop feeling guilty about it. There are times when we don't have the emotional bandwidth to be there for anyone else. Putting ourselves first in that instance isn't selfish. Self-care benefits us, as well as anyone else around us.

We have the right to bring self-care into our daily habits, just like taking a shower, putting on deodorant, and brushing our teeth. We must recognize that when we neglect our mental well-being, our physical health can be directly impacted and vice versa.

Supporting a loved one through a mental health crisis can be exhausting, but learning to leave room for moments of joy and laughter is like the sun breaking through the clouds.

**EXERCISES FOR SELF-CARE AND WARDING OFF BURNOUT**
Even if you feel you're good at self-care, I invite you to kick it up a notch!

1. What would your perfect day of self-care look like?

2. Journal your self-care activities, or sign up for some apps that provide calming meditations or support keeping track of your exercise, the number of steps you take in a day, your breathing, heart rate, etc.

3. Make a list of things you find yourself doing for others and a list of things you do for yourself. Are your lists balanced, or do you need to make an adjustment and do more for yourself?

4. What are some of the ways you already practice self-care? Feel free to add your own methods for warding off burnout.

5. Put an action plan together for when and how you plan on practicing self-care. The world is full of good intentions, so don't just talk about it. Do it! You'll thank yourself.

Chapter Eight

# Cultivating Resilience

Meet Charlene. We've been friends for more than 30 years. I met her back in the 1990s when a mutual friend of ours connected us, and we've been blessed to be friends ever since. We've witnessed each other's stages of life, including the challenges.

Charlene has a background in law enforcement, and she believes her training instilled resilience in her that she's been able to use in daily life dilemmas. After retiring, she became a certified resilience coach.

When she put her resilience program into practice, she discovered its healing benefits on her brain and overall wellness. She gained a greater awareness outside of her responder silo and realized the importance of resilience in everyone.

Our friendship has come full circle from giggles, travel, and now mentors working on various projects together. I asked Charlene to share her experience with navigating her loved one's mental well-being decline and how the practices she put in place continue to build her "resilience muscles" despite adversity.

She put it this way:

*Watching a loved one's mental well-being decline may just be one of the toughest adversities life can throw you. Loved ones hold so much influence over us, good and bad, and when they suffer, we generally follow suit—hence the contagion. In my instance, there was no decline. It was a sudden, needless act of sanctuary trauma that knocked my husband out at the knees. Sanctuary trauma is when the very organization that employs you and is expected to support you . . . treats you poorly and abuses their authority, creating an unsafe workplace. In the first responder world, this can mean the difference between life and death.*

*As first responders, we dealt regularly with the known risks and managed our operational stress injuries daily. Yet, I was not prepared for what happened to us. In 2021, in one crucial moment, his management team made a near fatal leadership choice that left the strongest man I know crumbling to the ground—physically and mentally. This has left scars not only on him, but on me, and our now two teen children.*

*Despite my desire to crumble, too, I knew it was on me to keep our family functioning, and it was going to be for a long time. My husband's heart and soul were torn out when he was robbed of his firefighter identity, and he was left to navigate the mental health repercussions, which influenced our entire household. I knew I needed to dig deep, and I was in for a marathon. So I embarked on formalizing my resilience coaching, where I not only earned my certification, but I brought awareness to many practices that I have used to strengthen myself.*

In this chapter, we'll talk about some of the practices that helped Charlene deal with such an emotionally and physically difficult situation. We'll work on strengthening your resilience, too, so that you can handle the tough moments when they come.

### What Is Your "Why"?

Charlene says we all need a reason why we want to cultivate greater resilience—a reason that makes us want to do the work of becoming stronger. Digging deep and reflecting on your "why" will keep you hanging on when life gets tough. And when you're navigating a loved one's mental health decline, life can get very tough.

Charlene tells people that their "why" should make them cry. It should be powerful and important. For her, it was the desire to keep her family together, including her two teens, while her husband was dealing with his challenges.

She emphasizes that as human beings, we're hard-wired for comfort, but there's nothing comfortable or easy about mental health struggles. So she worked hard to change her habits, which in turn strengthened her resilience. "Changing habits takes repetition, failure, and more repetition for them to stick," she says.

No matter the cause of our loved one's mental health decline, it's vital that we grow our resilience in order to be happier and healthier.

## The Resilient Mind/Body Connection

The art of being resilient stems in part from the activities of our mind, body, and spirit. First, we'll focus on the physical and mental factors at play. Many of our behaviors and emotions arrive instinctively and by default, so let's dive into the roles that our mind and body play in terms of our ability to be resilient in times of challenge.

*The Amygdala.* This small part of the brain processes our emotions, but if it doesn't function properly, it can wreak havoc with our feelings and behaviors, causing undesirable symptoms.[1]

A big component of resilience involves strengthening our amygdala. It has taken me years to do it, and it's an ongoing practice to keep my responses to challenging situations as healthy as possible. When navigating a loved one's mental illness, having a good idea of the amygdala's function will help you maintain emotional well-being.

The amygdala plays a vital role in our fight, flight, freeze, or fawn responses. These responses are meant to help us protect ourselves when faced with a perceived threat in our environment. Essentially, when we feel threatened, we either fight to protect ourselves, flee to protect ourselves, or freeze like a deer in the headlights. Fawn is a lesser-known response in which we might do whatever the person threatening us wants in order to keep ourselves safe.

These responses aren't necessarily bad if they keep us from harm. The problem is that our amygdala often goes into these modes when it perceives a threat that isn't as dangerous as we think or perhaps that doesn't even exist at all. For example, someone might make what they

---

1. Cleveland Clinic, "Amygdala," last reviewed April 11, 2023, accessed January 23, 2025, https://my.clevelandclinic.org/health/body/24894-amygdala.

consider to be an innocuous comment, but we take it as an insult, which throws our amygdala into high gear. It then causes us to react by fighting back, running away, freezing and feeling anxious, or fawning. Making our amygdala more resilient requires awareness to assess when it causes us to overreact. Then we can stop and make a choice that brings reason into the picture. If, for example, someone makes a comment that feels hurtful, we might assess the situation and realize the person didn't mean it that way. Or perhaps they did, but we don't necessarily have to feel threatened by it.

We can also reduce symptoms of anxiety, improve emotional regulation, and promote overall well-being by practicing the calming exercises we discussed in Chapter 7, such as meditation, decluttering of the mind, and deep breathing.

***Our nervous system.*** Perhaps you've said or been told, "you're getting on my nerves." Although no one can literally "get on" our nerves, it describes the feeling when our emotions take over. Our parasympathetic nervous system controls our heart rate and immune system, as well as our ability to rest and digest our food. These functions are involuntary, so we can't control them consciously. High levels of stress and anxiety can overstimulate our parasympathetic nervous system and lead to vomiting, dizziness, and abdominal pain. In other words, our body reflects our mind, proving that there's a direct connection between them.

***What happens in vagus.*** The vagus (or vagal) nerve is actually a set of nerves in our parasympathetic nervous system. If we stimulate this set of nerves, we can calm our nervous system.

A common way to stimulate the healthy function of the vagus nerve is through deep belly breathing; I like to refer to this as the "Buddha belly breath." Do this by breathing in slowly through your nose, fully filling your belly with air until you feel a slight abdominal stretch. Then release the breath slowly through your mouth.

There are many kinds of breathing exercises that can help you shift your focus away from stress. Your mind processes one thing at a time, so when you focus on the inhale and exhale of your breath, you can't focus at the same time on what's making you feel anxious.

Another form of breathing that can significantly affect the regulation of the nervous system and vagus nerve during high stress and anxiety comes from the natural wisdom of babies, called the "infant sigh." Think of an upset infant. They often take two sharp inhales and a long exhale. Doing this is one of the fastest ways to reset your fight or flight response and calm your nervous system.

These breathing techniques also slow down our heart rate and relax our body. The moment we anticipate any kind of stress, most of us hold our breath. So the saying, "take a breather," isn't just an off-the-cuff statement. There's validity to its power.

Stop right now, and check in with your body. Scan it from the top of your head to the tip of your toes. Are you holding tension anywhere? For example, once when I was at a funeral, my back started to tense up. I realized that out of stress and grief, I was standing there the entire time with my butt cheeks squeezed tightly, which triggered my sciatica. I had to shift positions and move my body to release the hold and tension. Remember that healthy movement boosts the brain's feel-good hormones, such as dopamine and serotonin. Staying in one position for a long period of time can have an adverse effect on the body and mind, increase lethargy, create sleep issues, and heighten our stress levels. So take that five-minute break to get up and walk around, perhaps switching from a sit-down position to standing and stretching.

When we become more aware of what's happening with our body, we're less likely to activate the amygdala, which keeps us on high alert with stress hormones flooding the body. Here are some more ways to encourage a calm nervous system and stay out of fight/flight/freeze/fawn mode:

1. Slow down. Are you always on the go? Do you sometimes get from point A to B without remembering how you got there? Or are you always rushing to get somewhere at the last minute, not giving yourself ample travel time between calls and meetings? Slow down, and be more mindful of your surroundings. When you move too fast, your brain goes into task mode, which automatically puts your amygdala on high alert and keeps your nerves on edge.

2. Be mindful of how often you reach for your phone. Do you take breathers from it, or do you check it constantly? I've been working on this myself, especially while writing this book, and I can notice a big difference. I discovered how often the phone distracts me, so I started to use its Do Not Disturb function.

3. Express and process your stress as it happens. When you ignore your emotions, they become stuck. Then it's harder to get out of fight, flight, freeze, or fawn mode.

## Red, Yellow, Green, Go!

A few years ago when COVID-19 was at its peak, the demand for mental health training became overwhelming. As a result, I was on the fast track to burnout. I scheduled back-to-back trainings, sometimes a few in the same day!

Packing your schedule with very little time for rest or reflection can quickly lead to chronic stress. It puts your nervous system into overdrive. Naturopath Dr. Hilary Chambers shared a tool with me that has helped me immensely. It's a metaphor for traffic lights. Red is for the most intensely stressful events, either physically or emotionally. Yellow is for moderately intense events, while green is for easy events. I make sure I don't schedule red events close to each other, and when I know one is coming up, I prepare for it in advance with self-care. (Of course, this only works with events we have planned, not with stressors that happen unexpectedly. But that's when our work on resilience comes into play! And the more we reduce our stress from planned activities, the more resilient we'll be for the unexpected.)

When you're creating your schedule, be mindful of the level of energy, stress, and/or mental capacity each item will require. Label them by the traffic light colors so that you can schedule accordingly. What you consider red, yellow, or green will be unique to you, however.

For example, a red event for me is showing up for virtual or in-person meetings, keynote speeches, teaching, or traveling. Although I enjoy doing these "red" events, I recognize the amount of physical and emotional resources they take. Yellow events could be social, sporting events, or personal and professional appointments. Green could be hobbies, forms of self-care, rest, or time spent with a friend or loved one.

Try to spread your most stressful tasks/events over the week rather than trying to tackle everything on a Monday. Sometimes, of course, it will be impossible to prevent too many red or yellow events in a row. But knowing that they're red and yellow will allow you to schedule in rest time as soon as possible. The intention is to avoid making a habit of too many red and yellow events scheduled together without some green in between.

## Emotional Maturity

Back in the late 1990s, I had difficulty managing my emotions and life's ups and downs. It affected my work life and relationships. I worried that I might be diagnosed with a mental health disorder just like my mother. Her colleague referred me to the top psychiatrist in Toronto, so I met with him several times and shared the symptoms I was experiencing. I was overly sensitive, angry, crying frequently, and struggling to sleep. I had a feeling of emptiness, victim mentality, lack of self-worth, and my mind raced with negative thoughts. On my last visit with him, he said, "Yvette, you are so normal. What you're going through is what we call emotional maturity—'growing pains.'"

Emotional maturity happens gradually, and we have to go through a lot of growing pains along the way. But we also need to make a concerted effort to become more mature. I knew, for example, that I needed to equip myself with the tools to handle stress better, make thoughtful decisions, and maintain a positive outlook. Without emotional maturity, we aren't resilient enough to cope with the sometimes volatile and erratic ups and downs of our loved one's symptoms.

Unlike puberty, there's no age range for emotional maturity. It can happen at any stage in life and is often prompted by circumstances where resilience is required. One of the reasons I became a psychotherapist was because of what I'd been through in my life. As a result, I recognized the value of emotional maturity. I realized that how I managed my emotions directly impacted how I showed up in the world for myself and others, so I knew I wanted to help other people who struggled with the same issues.

## Self-Awareness

Building resilience relies a lot on self-awareness, which is an understanding of our thoughts and emotions, as well as how they affect our actions.

Let's acknowledge the fact that you're reading this book, so you have a certain level of self-awareness because you *know* you're reading this book. You're also aware that you need support while navigating through your loved one's mental well-being decline. But stop to notice what you're actually thinking. What is your internal dialogue?

Sometimes, we are our own worst enemy. We say things to ourselves in our mind that we would never say to a friend or loved one. Are your thoughts healthy for you, or are they making you unhealthy? I invite you to be mindful of what you say to yourself, and challenge negative thinking if it starts to develop. That negative thinking can do much to undermine your resilience.

For strategies on changing negative thinking, cognitive behavioral therapy (CBT) is very effective. For example, CBT can help you discover what emotions and thoughts lead you to behave in certain ways. Think about a time when you acted in a way that surprised you or that you regretted. Did you understand why you acted that way? If not, that's a gap in your self-awareness. When you're more aware of why you do what you do, you can make changes to avoid regretful or hurtful actions. Of course, none of us is 100 percent self-aware, and it's an ongoing task to learn more about ourselves and our underlying motives.

One common habit of human beings that gets in our way is the tendency to "make things mean things" that they don't actually mean. Remember the innocuous comment that sent the amygdala into overdrive? That's an example of making something mean what it might not mean at all. Here are more examples: When a child falls and scrapes their knee, the child's mother might automatically think, "I'm a terrible mother!" If your boss calls you into their office for a meeting, you might immediately assume, "I'm getting fired!" But then you get a promotion instead. If your partner doesn't text you back right away, you might automatically think they're breaking up with you when it's just that their phone battery died. All of these can cause us to quickly move into fight/flight/freeze/fawn mode.

It may be human nature to jump to conclusions, but it only activates our amygdala and puts us on high alert for no good reason. It's a variation on the "what if" thoughts we've previously discussed. It's a kind of "catastrophizing," which is a response to previous traumas in which something has hurt or frightened us. That's why the amygdala is on high alert. But just because something painful happened in the past doesn't mean situations will always go wrong. Therefore, self-awareness is necessary in order to recognize these thoughts so that we can stop ourselves from assuming the worst.

If this is a problem for you, I highly recommend seeing a CBT therapist or finding a CBT program online. They'll help you reframe unhelpful thoughts so that they are healthier, more balanced, and more flexible, which will in turn positively affect your behaviors and increase your resilience. It doesn't necessarily mean your fears will go away entirely, but instead of jumping to conclusions, you'll be more likely to say, "I'm afraid of what might happen, but I also know I have the skills to manage it." That's what self-awareness can do for you and how it can help you become more resilient.

### EMOTIONAL REACTIONS VS. RESPONSES

How many times have you had a knee-jerk reaction and regretted it later? Think of a mosquito bite. When you scratch, it just gets itchier and maybe even starts to bleed. When you don't scratch it, the need to scratch starts to dissipate. That's when healing begins.

This is an example of the difference between *reacting* and *responding*. Scratching is reacting, while not scratching is responding. When the situation is emotional, responding is a particular skill that requires a lot of practice. Again, *reacting* happens naturally because it's instinctive, while *responding* requires thought and the self-awareness we just discussed, which takes more time.

As author/speaker Brad Stulberg has put it: "When you react to a situation, you fuse with it and become it. Going from one reaction to the next is an emotional rollercoaster. When you respond to a situation, however, you put a few degrees of freedom between a deeper and more stable sense of self and the ever-changing current of your life."

When we learn to respond rather than react, we promote greater resilience because we have an attuned skill for handling conflict.

Since the amygdala is the more primitive, instinctive part of the brain, it processes our emotions and takes charge quickly, focusing on our survival and fast responses to threats. This is what happens when we have a knee-jerk reaction. When we *respond* instead of react, we activate the prefrontal cortex part of the brain that connects us to social behavior and the ability to make more sound decisions. This is why they say to never make a major decision while feeling emotional. When we take our time, our nervous system can calm down. Then we can weigh options, think about consequences, and make choices based on reason rather than emotion.

Of course, this is great in theory, but when we're in the throes of fight mode, we have a strong impulse to react and protect ourselves. That's when we must learn to take a breath, remind ourselves not to take anything personally, and say, "I need a moment to think about that" or "let me digest what you're saying before I respond."

Another way to avoid reacting too quickly is to press your tongue against your two front teeth while the other person speaks. It will help ground you, keeping you in the present, as your tongue remains still regardless of how much your mind might be spinning.

Cultivating a habit of responding thoughtfully can lead to fewer arguments and more empathetic/compassionate resolutions to conflict. When you're getting ready to respond, here are some questions that will guide your thought process:

*How am I feeling right now?* Acknowledge how you feel. Does the reaction you're having match what's happening? As in the examples already mentioned, sometimes the situation triggers something from the past, and we overreact because our amygdala determines there's more of a threat than actually exists. For example, someone might make a joke that sounds as though they're questioning your intelligence. It triggers an extremely hurtful experience you had with a teacher who told you that you're stupid. So you react angrily to the person in the moment, but your reaction is really for the teacher of the past. Taking the time to respond rather than react so that you can access your self-awareness will be key to assessing whether your feelings are connected to what's happening in the moment or to a previous experience or belief.

*What are your intentions?* As you prepare your response to the situation, get clear on your intentions. Are you looking to "win," resolve the conflict, bring closure, set a healthy boundary, communicate a point, or offer further support? Have you evaluated whether you have any negative preconceived notions of what the other person is thinking or feeling? When my mind starts running away with what they "*could* be thinking," my dad tells me to say to myself, "don't go there." I find this is a great phrase to repeat to myself when my mind starts to spin in an unhealthy way.

*How can you express your feelings in a healthier way?* Resist the urge to overanalyze, blame, or argue things "tit for tat." If you are met with combativeness, don't engage. Perhaps pick a time when cooler heads prevail. Let the person discuss their points first. As discussed in Chapter 5, listen and communicate non-judgmentally. Look for ways to love and accept the other person as you manage your expectations. Think about how you can communicate your feelings in a way that's honest yet respectful. The goal is to share your thoughts with clarity and calm so as to avoid escalating the argument.

*Do you have all the information?* Problems tend to occur as a result of misunderstandings. Do you have the information you need to make an informed response? Ask questions rather than assume, and come from a place of curiosity rather than fix-it mode. Keep your focus on the issue at hand. Seek to understand. You might say something like, "I recognize that this is upsetting. Please help me understand what's going on."

The key takeaway here is to lengthen the time between your reaction and your response. The more you practice this, the healthier it will be for you and your loved ones.

## Emotional Anchoring

Emotional anchoring is another helpful tool that promotes resilience when we'd like to feel differently than we currently feel. It can bring calm and comfort. Emotional anchoring is like having a special person ready any time we need a warm hug.

You may already anchor your emotions without realizing it. Have you ever heard a song that brings a smile to your face? There are two songs that come to mind for me. One is "Take Me Home, Country Roads" by John Denver. As I previously mentioned, I had surgery for basal cell carcinoma on my nose. As they started the surgery, that John Denver song came on in the background. To me, it sounded like he was singing "country ROSE." The music was streaming in and out, very loud and at times soft. The surgeon asked what was happening with the music volume. I said, "I know why." But when the surgeon asked me to clarify, I said, "I can't say because it will make me cry." That's the last thing I wanted to happen during surgery on my nose!

After the surgery, she said, "Okay, tell me now." I explained that my mom had died of breast cancer about five years before, and roses were of spiritual significance for her. I felt she was letting me know that she was there to bring me comfort. Even though my surgery was nothing compared to my mother's breast cancer operation, it was still triggering for me to have any type of cancer.

The surgeon validated my feelings and comforted me. "Your mom is definitely here," she responded. We joked how the experience also showed that there was nothing subtle about my mom! Now, I think of my mother and that day every time I hear the song, so it's an "anchor" that helps me shift my emotional state. If I need that anchor, all I have to do is play that song.

The second anchoring song for me is "Chiquita" by Abba. It was my mother's favorite. A few months after she died, I woke up with the song in my head. I took it as a sign from her that I would be okay. So again, the song always reminds me of my mom and comforts me, pulling me out of a negative emotional state.

Fast forward to a few weeks ago over breakfast with Dave. I told him that I haven't been feeling the same level of excitement about life as I did before my mother's death. I wondered if I'd ever feel that deep excitement again. Later that day, I went to an appointment, and "Chiquita" started playing over the waiting room speaker. I then thought, "I wonder what would have happened if that song had come on instead of 'Country Roads' during my surgery." Believe it or not, the very next song to play was "Take Me Home, Country Roads!" After that, all the music stopped completely.

When I'm in need of comfort, I play these songs or sing them in my head. In an instant, it feels like a kiss from my mom in heaven, and I'm comforted.

You can also anchor a positive emotion by holding a rock or crystal. Close your eyes, and tap into a feeling of comfort, support, or whatever calms you. By anchoring it into the rock/crystal, when you need comfort or want to change your emotion, pick up that rock to take you to the feeling you want. You can do the same with scents (flowers, essential oils), a rubber band on your wrist, charms, a particular physical position, or visualization in your mind's eye. You choose!

## Managing Emotions

Anchors like the ones we just discussed help us manage our emotions, and resilience has a lot to do with learning how to manage them, especially when they're particularly intense. Even so, the intensity isn't necessarily the problem. What we do with the emotion is the problem. Of course, as I've said, the key isn't to numb, ignore, or judge what we feel.

Instead, think of surfing your emotions as though they are a wave, instead of being swept away and drowned by them. And stay aware of what you say to yourself about them. Are you critical of yourself and/or the emotion? Would you speak to a loved one the same way? When the emotions surface, have some grace and compassion for yourself and what you're going through. Remind yourself that all emotions are temporary. Little will promote resilience more than supportive, positive self-talk. As you practice it more and more, it will gradually become the voice that guides both your emotions and actions.

Here are some ways you can release the energy of an intense emotion:

*Get physical.* Move your body, stretch, bounce a ball, skip, putter around the house, garden, or blow bubbles.

*Change your environment.* Move to another room, or go outside and take a deep breath. Sometimes, changing your outer perspective can also change your inner perspective.

*Get destructive in a healthy way.* Rip the pages out of an old book, punch a pillow, or pop bubble wrap. Visit a rage room where people go to release stress by destroying furniture, appliances, and smashing plates against the wall. Scream, as we discussed in Chapter 7!

*Get creative.* Paint, color, crochet, knit, journal, or create a scrapbook, collage, or vision board.

*Bake.* Knead that dough, smash those potatoes, or whip those eggs.

*Visualize.* I highly recommend a life-transforming book called *Creative Visualization* by Shakti Gawain, a pioneer in the field of personal development for more than forty years. Creative visualization is the art of using mental imagery and affirmations to produce positive changes in your life.

*Get support.* We've already discussed therapy, but you could also join a group or club to gather with people of similar interests.

*Acupuncture.* This is a practice of traditional Chinese medicine. Tiny needles are inserted very superficially into the skin at particular points to stimulate the nervous system and promote physical and emotional healing. I've been getting acupuncture for years, and it's been life-changing in helping me manage my emotions.

*Social media.* Sometimes, social media gets a bad rap, but depending on how you use it, these sites and apps can be supportive. When I shared about my skin cancer diagnosis, I received overwhelming sentiments of love and support that helped me process my emotions.

*Give back.* Try volunteering and contributing to others. It can help you move through your emotions and heal.

## DEADHEADING

Deadheading is a process of pruning old growth and seed heads from a plant to promote new growth and reflowering. It gives the plant more energy to create, and it often grows thicker and fuller than before. Leaving dead flowers and leaves depletes the plant and may even cause it to struggle to survive.

We can deadhead our lives, too! It's not only beneficial but crucial for our mental health. To do this, we eliminate what brings us down, actions that no longer serve us, foods that react poorly with our body, and financial obligations that aren't necessary. You may even need to let go of people with whom you are no longer in alignment or at least limit time with them.

The company you keep matters and will help you enormously when you need to call on your resilience. When you have the right people in your inner circle, you're able to be authentic and feel safe psychologically and emotionally. Around these people, you should feel no need to shrink yourself, dim your light, or put up a façade. This can give you extra strength, especially when times are challenging.

In short, what are you "subscribing" to that might be harming you or at least not helping you? Self-care involves "unsubscribing" to all things that don't align with your growth, contribute to your peace, or make you happy.

Note, however, that when you deadhead a plant, it may look a bit droopy and sparse at first. Similarly, you'll likely go through a period of adjustment after deadheading your life. It might feel scary or lonely. You may worry you've made a mistake. But it's all part of cultivating resilience. Just know that deadheading helps you regulate your emotional safety and make room for healthier situations, new growth, and the opportunity to flourish.

## HELLO, GOD—IT'S ME, YVETTE

My intention for this section is to provide spiritual encouragement, hope, and faith for the challenges you may face while loving someone through a mental illness. Please take what you wish from this section. If you feel it doesn't apply to you, feel free to skip it.

Shortly after my mom died, I was sitting with a couple of friends, and the topic of God came up. One of them explained why there's no God. I stopped her and said, "Please stop. I don't know for sure there's a God, but my belief in a God or higher power is the only thing keeping me here right now on this earth. Please don't try to take that away from me." I didn't have suicidal thoughts, but in my grief, I was hanging on by a thread. The hope and faith that there was something bigger gave me comfort.

For example, my young niece, Isabelle, was searching for her Elf on the Shelf named Tommy but was in a panic because she couldn't find him. Adorably, she thought he'd gone back to the North Pole. I told her she needed to *believe* he was there. With her belief creating a new attitude, she found him. My hope for you is that like Isabelle, you will have hope and faith that you matter and that you aren't alone. Have faith that when you need support, it will show up for you in many ways such as through prayer, in people, in coincidences, in serendipity, in blessings, in gratitude, in a book, or in a song.

I recently saw a post on Instagram by Sonia Choquette, a dynamic, globally celebrated spiritual teacher. I have been a fan of hers for more than thirty years. She has given me permission to share it with you here. It's a prayer for anxiety that was gifted to Sonia by angels ten years ago while she was on the Camino de Santiago in Spain, and it has never failed to bring her peace, grounding, and clarity. As you read it, let the words wash over you, and trust in the divine support that always surrounds you.

You are held. You are loved. And your prayers are always heard. Save this prayer for when you need it most, and share it with someone who might need a little extra light.

> *Holy Mother, Father God, loving light of the universe, please help calm my anxiety. Relieve all the tension and worry in my bones and allow me to place it in your loving care. Take the distress I now feel and help me transfer this free-floating worry and tension into confident faith to address everything that comes my way in a confident, grounded, peaceful manner. Thank you for your constant love and support and reassurance as I face the unknown, and I thank you with my whole heart and spirit for answering my prayer.*

### Food for Thought

Did you know food can have a significant impact on your mental health and resilience? One of my mentors, Julie Daniluk, holistic nutritionist and author of five award-winning and best-selling books, taught me about healthy foods she refers to as a "LIVEit" rather than a "DIEit." She helped me not only choose "feel good" foods, but gave me psychological support about my relationship with food.

I have since learned through personal experience that there's a direct connection between my body and emotional health. The foods I've chosen to eat have changed my chemical makeup.

Nutrient-based foods feed our body, brain, *and* emotions. As Julie taught me, eating refined sugars and flours inhibits the production of our brain's natural pleasure chemicals. Healthy whole foods are packed with the nutrition our brain needs to produce a positive, calm, and more alert state that leads to less stress.

When my mother was in the hospital for close to a month, Julie's nutritional instruction helped me keep my emotions balanced and gave me the strength to endure the marathon of what I call hell. Yes, I felt despairing at times, but eating a healthy diet helped me immensely. In the past, I would have drowned my worries and heartache in sugary treats, pizza, and burgers that would have only made me feel worse. I'm convinced I wouldn't have been able to cope if I'd done that.

My definition of "comfort food" has also changed drastically. The foods I choose now bring me true comfort with an added bonus of joy and vitality. And the more "feel good foods" I choose, the more I want them.

Here are some of Julie's nutrition suggestions that can support your mental health and build your resilience, helping you cope with crises and stress:

*Stabilize your blood sugar* by cutting down on refined sugar. Refined sugar makes us anxious and sad, and it causes neurological inflammation that compounds our stress. Try putting some nut butter on a date, for example. Eat raspberries, blueberries, strawberries, and other low glycemic fruits instead. These provide lots of vitamin C, which reduces the stress hormone cortisol. Blueberries are especially rich in vitamin C and have been studied as one of the best fruits to lower stress levels. Try making a smoothie with them!

*Stabilize your blood pressure* by enjoying unrefined sea salt. It's great on macadamia nuts or curry-covered cashews. The electrolytes help carry the electrical charge through your body so that your brain can function better. Plus, unrefined sea salt is scientifically proven to reduce cortisol levels. For those of you with high blood pressure, enjoy more avocados that provide potassium, which reduces blood pressure.

*Love your gut.* When we're stressed, our gut flora is stressed, too. Considering up to 90 percent of the serotonin feel-good chemical is made in our gut, we need all the good bacteria we can get! Reinstate good bacteria by eating fermented foods such as sauerkraut, coconut yogurt, or pickles, as well as taking probiotic supplements.

*Help your nervous system.* A person under stress burns vitamin C, making it crucial to resupply the body with it during times of stress. Besides the berries previously mentioned, red peppers are a great source of it. Greens are also very important, as they're full of B vitamins. Every B vitamin plays a specific role in our nervous system, and vitamins B6 and B9 are especially critical for helping our brain cope with stress. Broccoli sprouts are an amazing source of these and are generally easy to digest.

Of course, these foods are just suggestions, and you must make choices based on your body and any allergies or food sensitivities you have.

## Sleepy Time

Don't underestimate the power of sleep. It impacts everything, including your emotions. If your sleep is inconsistent, poor, or not long enough, it directly affects your parasympathetic nervous system's ability to reset. In short, it's impossible to be resilient without good sleep.

To maximize your healing sleep, follow these suggestions:

*Keep a consistent sleep schedule.* Get up at the same time every day, even on weekends or during vacations. Set a bedtime early enough to get at least seven hours of sleep.

*Establish a relaxing bedtime routine.* Turn off electronic devices at least thirty minutes before sleep, and limit exposure to bright light in the evening. Use your bed only for sex and sleeping.

*Make your bedroom quiet and relaxing.* Keep the room at a comfortable, cool temperature. When was the last time you got a new bed or flipped the mattress? Are your pillows supportive? Your bedroom is your sanctuary, so investing in the best bed, sheets, and pillows is an investment in many good nights of sleep.

*Watch what you eat and drink before bedtime.* If you're hungry at night, eat a light, healthy snack, not a heavy meal. Avoid caffeine in the late afternoon or evening. Perhaps have chamomile or lemon balm tea instead. Reduce your fluid intake before bedtime to avoid overnight or early morning trips to the bathroom.

*Exercise regularly, and maintain a healthy diet.* But don't exercise too close to bedtime!

## Juicy Bits

Self-care isn't just something you do when you're spent or on the verge of breaking down. To build your resilience, you must be proactive about it and determine what you personally need for your own health and well-being.

Strengthening your "resilience muscle" is of utmost importance when loving someone with a mental illness. Your quality of life depends on it. Remember that resilience includes your inner dialogue, so don't put yourself down. Although you may strive to do your best, you're also human.

When I spoke at an event not long ago, an audience member shared that he used to think this "self-care business was all malarkey." But then he had a life-changing experience and put self-care into action. He now says it made a world of difference in his life and the lives of his family members.

Preferably, you'll have several people you can turn to when times get tough. I hope and wish that for you. What we need most during challenges is an empathetic ear or another perspective.

No matter what you may be going through, the night will still turn into day and vice versa. The world keeps moving. There is comfort in knowing there are constants, despite the unpredictability. Believing in a higher power with faith, hope, and optimism can help along the way.

Whatever self-care practices you choose, they will help you give the best of yourself instead of just what's left of you. They won't save you from challenges, but they'll help you be better prepared and more resilient when those challenges arrive.

## Exercises for Resilience

1. Part of cultivating resilience is venting. Getting thoughts and feelings out of your mind and heart can help a lot. I invite you to write a letter to your loved one that you won't send, saying all the things you'd love to say but won't for fear of repercussions or hurting their feelings. Afterward, burn the letter, and as it burns, send it love, releasing your

emotions. Feel free to repeat this letter-writing practice whenever you need to get your feelings out.

2. Blow up a party balloon, and write in marker on it what you want to release. Perhaps you want to release resentment, fear, heaviness, anger, guilt, shame, the desire to fix, etc. Write as many things as you want, and then pop the balloon! Release the feelings with love and forgiveness for others and yourself. I invite you to journal what comes up for you during this exercise.

    When you're ready, blow up another balloon, and write all the things you desire for your relationship with your loved one. Perhaps you want peace, understanding, love, compassion, grace, healing, joy, giggles, etc. Take a picture of it so that you can look at it whenever you need reminding. When you're ready, pop that balloon, sending your wishes into the ethers. Journal about the experience.

3. Part of building resilience is protecting your peace at all costs. Make a list of ways you intend to do that. For example:

    I protect my peace by *implementing boundaries.*

    I protect my peace by *not engaging in drama.*

    I protect my peace by *responding when I'm mentally ready but not before.*

    I protect my peace by *making space for alone time.*

    I protect my peace by *taking time to respond rather than react.*

    I protect my peace by *discerning who is welcome in my inner circle.*

    I protect my peace by *managing expectations.*

    I protect my peace by *cultivating resilience.*

    *Now, add your own:*

    I protect my peace by _____.

    I protect my peace by _____.

# Epilogue: Climbing Your Mountain

As we end our time together, I want to share with you the story about my dad's "mountain."

He was born in Newcastle, Northern Ireland, where he lived until he was four years old. When he turned eleven, his father took him, along with some of his siblings, back "home." My dad remembers looking out his hotel window at Slieve Donard, the highest peak of the Mountains of Mourne. He begged his father to let him climb it, but clouds were in the way, making it too dangerous.

He was still determined to climb it, so at the age of sixty-seven, he managed to go back and do just that. He followed in his own father's footsteps, first making a pilgrimage to honor his family's legacy and the hardships his ancestors went through. He also did it to mark the next stage of his life. He had raised a family, was retired, and wanted to commemorate that significant time by finally climbing "his" mountain.

Then in 2022, at age fifty-three, I climbed what I affectionately call "my dad's mountain." It turned out to be a bigger experience than I imagined, teaching me lessons to last a lifetime. For example, I learned that climbing a mountain is similar to navigating through a loved one's mental illness. It requires preparation, knowledge, courage, endurance, determination, resilience, faith, hope, optimism, and more.

When you're preparing to climb a mountain or navigating through someone's mental well-being decline, it's imperative to take your own capacity into account. Are you at risk of harm? How can you best be in care of yourself under the circumstances?

While I never considered myself to be athletic, I had to prepare myself for the climb. I trained by walking up to eight kilometers a day, incorporating challenging hikes through forests and hills. I made sure I had the proper gear and a pair of walking sticks, which literally saved my life. I toughened up my feet by getting blisters and breaking in the special hiking boots my dad gave me. While you might not have to do physical training when dealing with mental health issues, it helps to learn as much as you can to prepare yourself for the challenges, which is what you've been doing while reading this book.

Before my climb, I got myself mentally ready by researching others' experiences, and I decreased my self-doubt by calming my mind chatter and increasing my positive self-talk. I surrounded myself with a support team of professionals, family, and friends—all things that are also important when dealing with someone's mental well-being decline.

I was motivated and determined to climb the mountain regardless of the challenges. I was ready. I was also blessed to have my partner, Dave, by my side. Through decades of working on my self-awareness, I knew the kind of support that would work best for me during the climb. As I wrote in Chapter 7, a key component to navigating someone's mental health symptoms is managing expectations. I had to do that before my climb, managing my own expectations, as well as Dave's.

I shared with him that the best way to support me was to NOT cheer me on. *You read that right!* You see, years ago, I did a long hike uphill in Tuscany, Italy. When I lagged behind everyone, a group member who had already finished came back to cheer me on. Although she meant well, the support was unsolicited and not suited to me. Even if it wasn't true, my internal chatter told me that she was "helping" only because I was an "inconvenience" in holding up the group and needed to be "fixed." This just added to the pressures I was already feeling.

Similarly, when your loved one is feeling overwhelmed or inadequate, they aren't necessarily looking to be fixed. Instead, they want to be accepted as they are. All I needed on that hike was a friend to walk alongside me as I completed the journey. In Chapters 4 and 5, I wrote about the ways we can best support our loved one while avoiding fix-it mode.

I was *aware* that for me, the mountain climb would be physically and mentally challenging. I *acknowledged* that I needed a different kind of support from Dave than I had received on that Tuscany hike. I *accepted*

## Epilogue: Climbing Your Mountain

that I would need help, and I needed to choose other *actions*. I wanted to take my time. I wanted to take away any pressures of time, "have-tos," or expectations. I vowed to be the tortoise, not the hare.

This might remind you of the four As (*Awareness, Acknowledgment, Acceptance, and Action = Change*) that you read about in Chapter 3. I knew I could climb the mountain, but focusing on *how* I was going to do it is what made the difference for me. As you climb your own "mountain," my hope is that the chapters in this book will provide you with the awareness, support, comfort, and instruction you need.

The climb took us close to nine hours, which is twice the average amount of time. About halfway up, we thought we were lost. Fear and doubt took over, and I didn't know if I'd have the strength to get back on track. Sometimes, in life, we feel like we're going down the "wrong" path, perhaps even going around in circles with no end in sight. We believe it may all be for nothing. Trust that even if you get diverted or go in the "wrong" direction, it's for your highest good. Learn from it, and move on.

Thankfully, we came across some fellow climbers who assured us we were on track and pointed us in the right direction. But that involved going up at a steep angle. We thought we might need ropes and spikes! From a distance, it looked almost impossible, but as we got closer, it wasn't as steep as we thought. Situations in life can feel like that, too. They may not be as impossible as they seem at first glance. Chapter 8 speaks to managing your emotions by changing your perspective.

When I told my fellow climbers that my dad—my inspiration—climbed the mountain when he was sixty-seven years old, they said, "Ah, so you're walking in your father's footsteps!" That's exactly what I was doing, fully aware of those who had gone before me. When I was halfway up the mountain, I even Facetimed with my dad, then age eighty-four. If you can find someone else who has been on a similar journey to yours, they can be your inspiration to help you keep going.

When we arrived at the saddle of the mountain, we met fellow climbers encouraging one another to continue the last leg to the top. It can bring us comfort if we recognize that each of us is surrounded by fellow "climbers" on our mental health journey. We're never alone.

## Epilogue: Climbing Your Mountain

Even though our climb was on a beautiful August day for those at ground level, the weather at the top of the mountain changed drastically, bringing billowing wind and sleet. Our mental health circumstances can also change like that at any given moment. You might feel joyful, hopeful, and optimistic when a dark cloud suddenly comes over you, changing your feelings instantly. I wrote about the factors that affect our mental health in earlier chapters.

When we reached the summit of the mountain, it was a cathartic release that made me sob. There were overwhelming tears of joy, gratitude, pride, and a feeling of sacredness. We did it! In awe and wonderment of how my dad managed it at age sixty-seven, I had to give him absolute RESPECT! It was August 3, which was also the third anniversary of my mother's death. I was literally in the clouds, so I felt closer to her.

We celebrated our accomplishment of getting to the top, ate some lunch, and made a video for my family to include them in the triumphant moment. When navigating a mental health crisis, it's also important to acknowledge our milestones and achievements, large or small. They'll be great reminders when times are tough.

When I started my descent back down the mountain, I took one look at the path and thought "Bloody hell! How am I going to do that?" I took it one steep step at a time. Then approximately one hundred feet down, I took a tumble and twisted my knee. Fortunately, I didn't do any major damage and was able to coach myself not to think of worse-case scenarios or engage with "what ifs." I wrote about anxiety and "what ifs" in Chapters 2 and 7. They can get in our way in any life situation.

At one point on my mountain climb, my hiking poles went flying. A young man retrieved them and handed them to me. "Do you need help?" he asked. I declined, noting that my partner, Dave, would assist if need be. The lad didn't try to fix me, make it all better, or watch my every move. He simply offered to help and carried on with his own journey. When there isn't an immediate risk and someone refuses your help, that's okay. It isn't personal, and it isn't your responsibility to make sure they're all right.

Despite having twisted my knee, I was able to continue my climb, even though it was painful. I did have to be especially careful of every step, and I had to use my left leg (the side that was prone to sciatica nerve pain) to carry most of the weight. Similarly, there are times when you need to lean on one person more than others. Who is that person for you? Acknowledge them for their unwavering support. Maybe send them a thank-you card. If you are that person for your loved one, take yourself out for a treat!

Dave was that person for me while I climbed the mountain. At times, of course, we supported each other. It was a great synergy, and I wouldn't have wanted to make that climb with anyone else. At one point, for example, there was a family of goats blocking our path, and Dave had no desire to go near them. He thought they would attack us. I looked to see if there was another route, but there wasn't. Sometimes, we need to forge ahead no matter how scared we feel. So I took a deep breath and started to walk toward the goats as I spoke to them in a loving voice. As we approached, they cleared the path for us.

When we finally got approximately five hundred meters from the bottom of the mountain, my knee was hurting a lot, and my legs felt like they would collapse. I started to feel afraid. It was then that I prayed to my mother for help. When you feel you have nothing left, pray, have faith, and hope that you WILL get through it. In Chapter 8, I wrote about a belief in prayer, which can bring comfort in our time of need.

Despite my pain, I dug deep and kept going down the mountain. Within minutes, the "mountain workers" came from behind on their own way down to go home. (Amazingly, they climb the mountain every day!) We had met and chatted with them a couple of times along our journey, so they were familiar with us. Realizing we had been on the mountain for quite some time, they stopped and asked how we were doing. I proceeded to tell them about my knee and wobbly legs, and they offered to drive us to the car park.

Without hesitation, I accepted the help this time! I have come to a point in my life of knowing my body/mind, so I knew instinctively to take the offer. Getting the ride to the car park meant I could bypass the forest we had hiked through to get to the bottom of the mountain, and it was not at all considered cheating. This allowed me to avoid further injury. So always remember that your safety is paramount, no matter what anyone else might say about it.

Do you know what supports are available to you? Will you wait until it's urgent, or will you accept help to avoid further injury or decline? When you need support, take it! Don't judge it; bless it.

When I finally got to the car and sat down, I cried an "ugly cry." It was such an emotional moment. I didn't know exactly what I was crying about. Was it the fact that I was safe after many scary moments? Were they tears for my accomplishment, gratitude for Dave, or tears for my mom or my dad and all those who came before me? It didn't matter. I didn't have to define or explain it. I felt those tears deep in my soul and let them flow. So remember that emotions need motion, even if you don't know why you're feeling as you are. Tears release feel-good endorphins that can ease both physical and mental pain.

Once we were back at our hotel, I propelled myself forward slowly down the hallway like a turtle, where we were greeted in our room by a bottle of champagne and afternoon tea that our friends, Kim and Eric, had gifted us. They opted to support us from afar, checking in on our mountain climb via text from the hotel spa. When you navigate your own "mountain," having an inner circle of trustworthy, supportive friends can make a world of difference. In Chapter 8, I wrote about the significance of being mindful of who or what you allow into your life as you cultivate resilience.

My mountain climb was a testament to my ability to overcome the odds. A few years prior to it, as I mentioned in Chapter 7, I had protruding disks pressing on my sciatic nerve. It was debilitating for sixteen weeks. At times, the pain was so bad that my legs weakened to the point of collapse. I needed a wheelchair, walker, cane, and helping hands.

There was a time when I thought I would never get better. My physical health affected my mental health and vice versa. If you had told me at that time that I would climb a mountain a few years later, I wouldn't have believed you. I had to put self-care into action to build my resilience muscles, and as a result, I no longer take being in care of myself for granted. Are you aware of your own capacity to withstand the side effects of your loved one's mental illness—the support, grace, and tenacity required? Even if you can't imagine having inner peace under challenging times, I'm here to tell you it's possible!

# Epilogue: Climbing Your Mountain

No matter where you are on your "mountain climb," I invite you to tap into your human ability to overcome, persevere, and go forward in courage.

## Because You Can

Back in 2017, I posted a video message on social media with the words, "because you can." When it comes to navigating yourself through your loved one's mental well-being decline, do what you *can* do. If you think something you want to do is impossible, it doesn't mean you can't do something else. Where in your situation can you do a "little" something, anything simply because you can?

My mom responded in the comment section to the post, writing: "very inspirational stuff, I am saying this because I can, quite often we come across difficulties in our lives that seem overwhelming, they can last a long time. We take it step by step towards the goal, never give up, I continue with my disabilities every day. I will never give up because I know I can reach the goal with the help of my prayers and tenacity!" I'm so grateful for those typed words of wisdom from my mother, especially after the hardships she endured.

It's a great reminder that we all have it within us to take it one step at a time. Little by little, we can make a difference for our loved one, while also taking care of ourselves. I wish you hope, and I pray that your loved one *will* come back "home" where they know they're loved and supported. And I send wishes that even though your circumstances may challenge you in many ways, you will maintain your own equilibrium and well-being.

# Acknowledgments

I'd like to start by acknowledging and giving thanks for the healing that took place for myself and my family while writing this book. I didn't realize the powerful impact this book would have on us. Although we all navigated a loved one's mental well-being decline, we each experienced it with our own unique perspective. Writing this book opened up a dialogue and gave us opportunities for healing on many levels.

Thank you to my father, who gracefully provided a safe space for me to share my experiences, diligently read through all the chapters, and provided his own insight. Right from the beginning, my dad has been a significant part of my support team.

I'm a firm believer that having a team of professional supports by your side can make a world of difference. Thank you to my soul sister, Kelly Goorts, R.Ac and founder of Pure Health, who has helped keep my mind, body, and spirit balanced for years. Thank you to Dr. Hilary Chambers, ND; Henry Janzen, RMT, DOMP; Dr. Sarah Adams (RIP); Dr. Mardi Charlton; and Julie Daniluk, RHN.

Thank you to all the professionals who helped my mom and other family members by supporting us while we navigated the mental well-being declines—especially Dr. Rufino Balmaceda and Dr. Rambir Bhatia.

Thank you to Samantha MacLeod, part of the MentalHealthTrainer.ca team who jumped in when needed, created time and space for me to write, and kept the "machine" running. Thank you to seoplus+, specifically Amanda Stephens and Brock Murray, who do a great job with our online presence.

## Acknowledgments

Thank you to my business partner, Tim Reinemo, who has cheered me on for many years, encouraged me to follow my professional dreams, and whom I fondly consider family.

Thank you to my personal editor, Melanie Votaw. You have such a beautiful way of conveying my written words succinctly. I'm sure the readers will appreciate it, too! Thank you for having my back and guiding the way.

Thank you to my book agent, Steven Harris. You were the first one to respond, and after our meeting, I knew you were the best fit. Thanks for believing in my vision and connecting me to my publisher.

Thank you to my publisher, Jonathan Kurtz, for recognizing the need for this book and for having faith in me.

Thank you to my inner circle of friends, specifically Linda Szenteszky (aka Marge), who has been with me every step of the way, as well as Kim Kovar, Eric Dionne, Brenda Saunders, Charlene Davidson, Alison Dove, Melissa Plunkett, Fareena Tsudek, Olga Nikolajev, and JOYanna Anthony. I feel so blessed to be surrounded by these special friends, who have made a significant difference in my life.

Thank you to my family. You have graciously listened to me speak "book language" for years, even when I repeated myself, especially Faith Murray. Your checking in and desire to read the book before it hits press was very encouraging to me.

A shoutout to all my UK family, specifically Eileen Murray and Alison Bartolo, who invited me to speak at their events and have contributed to many conversations about mental health. Thank you to Uncle Michael Wyeth for your candid shares and perspective. To my twin brother, Jonathan Murray (a.k.a. Jonny), we went through this experience together, a bond that will last a lifetime. Thanks for the almost daily calls and all your support and input. We are blessed.

To my significant other, David Succamore, thank you for being my foundation. Having you by my side through thick and thin has given me the courage to go forth in a brave new way.

And last but certainly not least, thank you to my mom. Thank you for being my forever cheerleader and encouraging me to write a book.

## Acknowledgments

You had faith in me before I did. Although our lives were challenging at times, I am so grateful to have had you as my mother. You are a big part of the empowered woman I have become. What I know for sure is that I am my mother's daughter.

In gratitude,
Love, Yvette

# About the Author

Yvette Murray is a psychotherapist (retired) in Toronto, Canada, and a facilitator of the Mental Health First Aid Certification, an evidence-based program available in more than thirty countries around the world. She is also a mental health advocate, influencer, and keynote speaker for nonprofit organizations, corporations, government agencies, and institutions. She is also a contributing author to the Mental Health Commission of Canada's *Catalyst* magazine.

Certified in Workplace Mental Health Law from Osgoode York University, Yvette offers coaching and training support on this topic. She has taught students employed by the Mental Health Commission of Canada, Global Affairs Canada, Canadian Federal Government, Canadian National Defense, Environment and Climate Change Canada, Scotia Trust, MD Trust, Scotia Wealth Management, EllisDon, Salvation Army, Shepherds of Good Hope, CFIA, UFCW, Loblaws, Starbucks, and various hospitals. These students have been from a variety of industries, including human resources, insurance, security, retail, law firms, banks, and many other trades.

In addition to her experience as a mental health educator, Yvette has experience with being a LivingWorks Instructor offering certified safeTALK Suicide Alert training, is a Certified LivingWorks ASIST Suicide First Aider, certified in safeTALK, and is a Suicide Alert Helper. She is also a Body Language Institute (BLI) Certified Instructor. A graduate of the BLI "You Can't Lie to Me" Train the Trainer program, she was mentored by the internationally sought-after body language expert Janine Driver—a *New York Times* best-selling author, award-winning keynote speaker, and the go-to expert in lie detecting and body language for the media, the FBI, CIA, ATF, and the International Chiefs of Police.

www.ingramcontent.com/pod-product-compliance
Lightning Source LLC
Jackson TN
JSHW020150220925
91348JS00002B/2